Good News for Your Autumn Years

Reflections on the Gospel of Luke

T. Josephine Lawler, OP

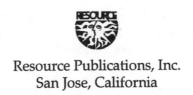

Resource Publications, Inc.
San Jose, California

A Leader's Guide to GOOD NEWS FOR YOUR AUTUMN
YEARS *is available for $7.95 through your bookseller or from
Resource Publications, Inc., at the address below.*

Editorial director: Kenneth Guentert
Managing editor: Elizabeth J. Asborno
Editorial assistant: Mary Ezzell

Photo on back cover taken by Anthony Marino

Reprint Department
Resource Publications, Inc.
160 East Virginia Street #290
San Jose, CA 95112-5876

Library of Congress Cataloging in Publication Data
Lawler, T. Josephine.
    Good news for your autumn years : reflections on the Gospel
of Luke / T. Josephine Lawler.
        p.   cm.
    Includes indexes.
    ISBN 0-89390-303-5
    1. Bible. N.T. Luke—Commentaries. 2. Ageing—Religious
aspects—Christianity—Meditations. I. Title.
BS2595.3.L385 1994
226.4′07′0846—dc20   94-21114

Printed in the United States of America

94 95 96 97 98 | 5 4 3 2 1

To my mother and father

Contents

Acknowledgments

I thank my God every time I
remember you, constantly praying
with joy in every one of my prayers
for all of you, because of your sharing
in the gospel from the first day until
now (Phil 1:3-5).

With Paul I give thanks for a number of
persons who have supported me in bringing
this work to completion. From the time of the
book's conception, Justus George Lawler, my
brother, has encouraged me and offered suggestions. Those with whom I have lived and
worked, as well as members of my own con-
gregation, have been patient and supportive.

I appreciate the words of endorsement of the book expressed by those who are so knowledgeable concerning its message: Eugene C. Bianchi, Evelyn Eaton Whitehead, and Sr. Loretta Wallauer, SBS.

I am grateful for the interest and painstaking editing of Kenneth Guentert and Elizabeth J. Asborno of Resource Publications, Inc.

St. Paul's expression of gratitude and mine apply in a special way to the remarkable women and men who have shared their own lives and thoughts so generously and sincerely during spirituality and aging sessions.

Preface

As older persons, we are embarking on a way of life that is new for us. While every phase of our lives had seemed new in its time, in the younger years others had gone before us who showed us how to live and many others had advised us. We, however, are the first large population to experience longevity. Every day some among us pass the hundred mark into very old age. Our older years may comprise as much as one-third of our lives; yet we have few models to guide us and few persons of experience to advise us.

As I pause on the threshold of my journey through my Autumn years, I frequently reflect on my present "young" older years and on the years to come. I share my reflections with you, my brothers and sisters, in the hope that this sharing may be helpful and may spark reflections of your own.

I am writing for two groups among us. First, for those of us who are not yet frail that we may have a spirituality of aging which undergirds our lives now and which will be our mainstay when we become weak, frail, and dependent. Secondly, I am writing for those of us who are now frail, in the hope that these reflections may enable a meaningful living of Jesus' way during our years of frailty, as we prepare for death and our entry into eternal life.

We are all aware of the possibility of frailty; nevertheless, a definition of *frail* as I use it may help. I consider a person frail who "is physically weak, sick, or disabled, and who needs assistance in order to implement simple daily living tasks."

I have selected the Gospel according to Luke for my reflections because Luke includes themes related to prayer, a way of life, and the role of the Spirit; because marginal people, such as the poor, women, and older persons, are emphasized (we older persons, especially those among us who are frail, may be marginal); because Luke, along with the other Gospels, presents the message of Jesus, and this message is the culminating message of God to all persons; moreover, because Luke presents the message of Jesus as a life of Jesus, thus enabling us to relate the message to our own lives.

Jesus did not and could not live every age, situation, and experience that persons after him would live, nor does salvation depend on his having so lived. Nevertheless, the incarnation and redemption, Jesus' way, are relevant to people of all ages and in all circumstances. Jesus' way is relevant, then, to all of us older persons. What we may need is an understanding of Jesus' message that is meaningful to us.

Luke's purpose was to tell Christianity's story to the world at large in order to attract converts and to gain respect for the new religion. He probably wrote in the 70s or 80s, when the Jews who survived the destruction of Jerusalem and of the Temple were striving to understand these events in terms of their relationship with Yahweh. At this time Judaism had influenced Christianity in such matters as the Mosaic Law and the way Christianity spread. Luke wrote in a church of gentile converts.

I have reviewed broad topical sections of Luke, with brief insights regarding suggested spiritual meanings of the texts for us as older persons. At times the insights apply to other populations or to people in general, as well as to us; these more general insights have been included because, in my experience, we may benefit from recalling them. We who have reached our Autumn years tend to have a lower self-image than we did during our early and middle adult years because of the loss of clearly defined "useful" roles in society; consequently, God's love for us, our inherent dignity, and the value of being, as well as of doing, are themes that need frequent emphasis with us.

The reflections in this work are often ordinary and mundane, just as Jesus' life and his teachings and reflections were often concerned with "ordinary" people and events.

Chapter One

John the Baptist and Jesus

*The Births and Hidden Lives
of John the Baptist and Jesus*

LUKE 1

1:1-4 / Prologue

The four brief verses of the prologue to the gospel introduce the two-volume work of Luke the evangelist—his gospel and the Acts of the Apostles. They testify to his intent to present a true account of events in the life of Jesus, events that culminated in the establishment of the Christian church.

We older readers reflect on Luke's account so that, like Theophilus, who is addressed in the prologue, we may know how well founded is Jesus' teaching. In reflecting on Jesus' teaching, we hope to follow his way, to embrace his values, and to be inspired to make the day-by-day decisions that stem from his way and values. In the complexity of our older years, we hope to discern with Jesus the decisions that enable us to live fully our remaining years and to die and rise, so that we may live forever with him.

1:5-25 / *The Birth of John the Baptist Foretold*

In reflecting on the gospel story of the birth and hidden life of John the Baptist and of Jesus, we might reflect also on our own birth, family heritage, and youth. Our reflection might lead to greater understanding of the influences of our period of youth on us as we are today and of the ways in which God has been with us as our lives unfolded, just as God was with John and with the boy Jesus. In fact, we might reflect on our total lives as a means of accomplishing what psychologists see as the tasks of the older years—finding meaning in life and achieving wisdom, maturity, and integrity.

The gospel begins during the reign of Herod the Great with God's coming through the mediation of an angel of the Lord to the elderly priest, Zechariah, while he was praying in the Jerusalem Temple. The angel announced that Zechariah's elderly, barren wife, Elizabeth, who like Zechariah was descended from the priest Aaron, would give birth to a son. The son would be filled with the Holy Spirit and, with "the spirit and power of Elijah," would go before the Lord "to make ready a people prepared for the Lord."

This announcement was especially important to Elizabeth as an older Jewish woman who until then had been childless, for childlessness was a condition looked down on by the Jewish people. We may be anxious because we have not achieved the life goals we had set and because we may feel useless in retirement. To God, however, we, like Elizabeth, are persons of worth who will be heard by God in our old age. Moreover, this last period of our lives, our older years, is a time of unique importance. It is that time when we may live especially close

to our God, who will call us at its completion
to follow in death and resurrection.

1:26-38 / *The Annunciation*

The annunciation of the birth of Jesus parallels the annunciation of the birth of John the
Baptist. Both follow the pattern of annuncia-
tions of births in the Hebrew Bible—the birth
of Isaac, Genesis 17:15-19; the birth of Samson,
Judges 13:3-20; and the virgin birth, Isaiah 7:10-
14. However, Luke 1:32-33,35,38, concerning
the annunciation of Jesus' birth, expands the
pattern. Luke seems to establish Jesus' divinity
(Jesus will be called "Son of God") while em-
phasizing the lowliness of Jesus' birth.

Having received reassurance concerning
her virginity that the Holy Spirit would "come
upon" her and the "power of the Most High"
would overshadow her, Mary, in her mature
youth, believed the surprising news that she
would bear the Son of God, Jesus. With the
little bit of information the angel gave and a
very uncertain and awesome future, Mary said
"Yes" to a heavy and frightening responsibility.

Reflection on Mary's readiness, on the angel's message from God, "Do not be afraid,"

4

and on the message, "The Lord is with you," may enable us as older persons to cope with the awesome uncertainty of our future mission as part of a burgeoning older population in a problem-plagued society. We might rely on the power of the Holy Spirit, who overshadows us, to strengthen us to pursue God's mission, even while that mission lacks clarity. Knowing that the Spirit is with us, we might take the small steps that we can discern.

As God's favored ones, we might accept the radical changes necessitated in our lives by our aging. Acceptance might replace angry or bitter responses to limiting changes. Thus we may receive God's way in the new and difficult—in moving into more limited and sheltered settings, in lifestyles imposed by chronic illnesses, in associating with nursing-home companions who irritate, or in relating to unfeeling caregivers.

1:39-45 / The Visitation

Mary's visitation to Elizabeth is the third event in Luke's infancy narrative and complements the other two events, the two birth announcements. The Mother of God went in haste to visit older Elizabeth. Because of the presence in Mary of her Lord, Elizabeth was "filled with the Holy Spirit," and the child in her "leaped for joy."

Mary's almost instant response with the news of Elizabeth's conception may remind us of the importance of our concern for others and our response to them during important occasions in their lives. Mary's visit and Elizabeth's response may affirm us in our efforts to reach out to family or neighbors who may need help and the presence of one who listens and cares.

We may be immersed within self because of physical limitations (poor hearing, visual losses, crippling arthritis) that render contact with the outer world an extraordinary effort. Concerned about a future with increasing limitations and illness, we may need to exert extra energy in order to focus on others.

No doubt during Mary's prolonged visit, Elizabeth told a very receptive Mary the entire story of the angel's announcement to Zechariah and Elizabeth's own pregnancy of over five months. Those of us who are frail shut-ins may have outlived close friends or spouses to whom we could speak unrestrainedly. Yet, we, like all persons, need to objectify our thinking in order to discern decisions we must make. We might take the initiative to ask a communion minister or a friendly visitor to plan time during the next visit for us to discuss some important topics. If we have no one to whom to turn, we might write our concerns prayerfully as a letter or conversation with Jesus (perhaps in a prayer journal).

1:46-56 / The Magnificat

Elizabeth marvels, "Why has this happened to me, that the mother of my Lord comes to me?" (In Jewish thought of that time, a woman's greatness was measured by her children.) She declares Mary most blessed among women. Mary, who echoes Hannah, mother of Samuel, sees the lowly and hungry in herself and knows and proclaims that God the Savior is glorified in her.

Her Magnificat reminds us that God values lowly ones, that mercy is for those who fear God rather than for those who revere great personages, and that God responds to those in need rather than to popular persons, who receive from many. In fact, Mary's hymn of praise sings of the dignity and glory of the *so-called* lowly (for none of God's people is lowly). The Magnificat alerts us to the privilege of being with the needy and lowly, perhaps in the person of a frail relative or neighbor. By preference we might respond to the lowly who are in need.

Mary reflected God's glory precisely because of her lowliness. In so doing, she foreshadowed her son, Jesus, whose life would be lowly and who would be savior of the lowly, thus reversing society's values.

Precisely because of our lowliness, weakness, and vulnerability, therefore, we reflect God's glory, for God, in mercy, looks upon the lowly and exalts the lowly with might. God's greatness has been manifested in love for us, in entrusting to us love and service of others, in allowing us to communicate the Savior's message and way. Believing in our God-given greatness and dignity, let those of us who are active seek a ministry of service to persons in need—to the lowly who have been exalted by God. Then, realizing God's glorification in us, we might pray in a hymn of praise like Mary's,

> My soul proclaims the greatness
>   of the Lord
>   and my spirit exults in God my
>   savior

because God has looked upon me, a
   declining aging servant.

Yes, from this day forward
   all generations and those who
      know me will call me blessed,
for the Almighty has done great
   things for me.

Holy is God's name,
   and God's mercy reaches from
      age to age
for us who know and fear God.

God has shown power.

God has routed pride of heart.

God has pulled down the
   independent from their
      self-sufficiency
and exalted the frail and powerless.

Those hungry for a fulfilling life, God
   has fulfilled;
those hungry with the good life, God
   has emptied.

God has come to the help of us
    elders, mindful of mercy—
according to the everlasting promise
    of mercy to the Son
    and his followers forever.

1:57-66 / The Birth and Circumcision of John the Baptist

Scholars note that naming a son after a family member was not customary among the Jews; nevertheless, Luke's narrative reflects such a custom. As part of divine revelation, Luke's interpretation of this story contains messages for us. According to the text, the neighbors and relatives decided to call the child Zechariah. They could not ask Zechariah in his dumbness to tell them the name of the child, and they did not ask Elizabeth. When Elizabeth, the mother, maintained that the child should be named John, they went to Zechariah. Writing the name "John," Zechariah upheld Elizabeth's decision (and obeyed the angel).

Elizabeth bore a son. The birth of a child is always wonderful, but her age rendered it doubly a miracle. When Zechariah named their son

John, as directed by the angel, he could speak again. What fulfillment for Elizabeth and Zechariah! How wonderful for the child that he was treasured as a child of promise!

The birth of the son was a miracle. But Zechariah's speech did not return at that moment. It returned when Zechariah fulfilled the angel's command and named the boy John. The great moments in our lives are when we say "Yes" to God's directions, when we will a response. These are moments greater than the miracles of life and death, over which we have no control. Our intent might well be to say "Yes" to all God wants of us.

1:67-79 / The Benedictus

God fulfilled the promise to Zechariah even though Zechariah questioned the angel's astounding, unexpected message. As we age, we tend more and more to think according to fixed patterns. We feel at ease within our patterns and resist changing them, even when they are disrupted by such circumstances as a broken hip. When permanently incapacitated, we may still insist on impossible schedules and residence in a home that was too large to maintain before the broken hip.

God understands our fears and resistance to new thinking, just as God understood Zechariah's questioning. Zechariah experienced dumbness as a result of his resistance and as a sign of God's displeasure. We may find ourselves incapable of articulating to our children and friends why, at the present time, we cannot change. Our faithful God, who kept the promise of a son to Zechariah, will support us and be faithful to us in our struggles to accept needed change.

The structure of Luke's infancy narrative indicates parallels between the birth, circumcision, and naming of John and the same events for Jesus, as well as parallels between Zechariah's Benedictus and the Magnificat, and the Benedictus and Simeon's Nunc Dimittis (2:29-32). Zechariah's Benedictus, which includes Hebrew Bible allusions, stresses continuity with God's promise to the Israelites. It is the link with the story of Jesus.

Like the older Zechariah, we, having reviewed the past and having reflected on the blessings in our lives as well as on the world around us, might consider God's faithfulness to us over the years. Rejoicing in God's presence with us in the past and now, we might pray, through the Spirit,

Blessed be the Lord, the God of the
    universe,
for God has visited us elders;

God has come to our rescue
    and has raised up for us
those who can save us in today's
    world,

even as God promised,
    by the mouth of Jesus and in
        Scripture from former times,
that God would save us from our
        enemies,
    from the hands of those
        who hate and would destroy
        us, the ill and weak.

Thus God showed faithful love to
    those who went before us;
thus God remembers the holy
        covenant,
    the Word God spoke to the
        Son, Jesus,
that God would grant us,
    free from fear,

to be delivered from terrorism in our
   streets and the nuclear
     threat,
to serve God in holiness and virtue in
   God's presence,
     all our days.

And you, young and old,
   God's children,
you shall be prophets of the Most
   High,
for you will go before the Lord
   to prepare the way for him,
   to give God's people
     knowledge of salvation
     through the forgiveness of their
     sins because of the mercy of
     our God,
who from on high will bring the rising
   Sun of justice to us,
to give light to us who live in
   darkness and the shadow of
     death
and to guide our feet into the way of
   peace.

1:80 / The Hidden Life of John the Baptist

That John the Baptist was born of older parents, who had the tolerance typical of grandparents, may have allowed him freedom of spirit. This freedom may have enabled him to mature and follow God's call and to live a lifestyle in the desert that was a departure from the usual lifestyle of his time.

We, who have been taught to understand the young by experience and wisdom gained over the years, might be encouraged by the story of John the Baptist to relate to the small children in our families. We might be the ones who consider the children and their thoughts important, who listen to them, and who cherish and love them. The children, then, like John, might gain the self-concept and confidence to follow God's way for them boldly.

LUKE 2

2:1-20 / The Birth of Jesus

How privileged we are that our Savior came as everyone does: as a helpless infant, full of beauty, hope, and promise, but unpretentious—born in poverty, with poor parents, and

without a home! This helpless infant ushered
into the world a way of life and of faith that
would revolutionize the whole western world.
Jesus, who said, "I am the way, and the truth,
and the life" (Jn 14:6), is truth and life through
his divinity and became the Way through the
mystery of his incarnation.

The infant Savior was known first by the
ordinary people nearby—the shepherds, who,
in spontaneous faith, went in haste to the manger in Bethlehem. Simple people, the shepherds were despised by the Jews, but Jesus
came for people in despised roles.

We, particularly those among us who are
frail, may sometimes feel that the young and
strong look down on us. That Jesus, who is the
Way, came into the world as a poor little one
and that he related to the despised and poor
may encourage us to seek and live Jesus' un-
worldly, poor way. Moreover, when we are
weak and can accomplish little, when we are
literally poor or in difficult circumstances, and
when the young and vigorous overlook us, we
may accept and value our unwanted way of life
because it resembles Jesus' life. Like the shepherds, we may glorify and praise God because
we have known the Savior.

2:21-40 / *Jesus Is Presented in the Temple*

A developmental task in old age is the achievement of integrity, whereby the older person accepts his/her own life and the people who have been part of his/her life. As we who are older read the story of Jesus' presentation in the Jerusalem Temple according to the Law of Moses, we may identify with the upright and devout Simeon, the old man in the Temple, to whom the Spirit revealed Jesus as Christ the Lord. Simeon accepted the revelation and accepted and rejoiced in Jesus as the promised one and the fulfillment of Simeon's life and of the Jewish people.

The time may come when we, like Simeon, can accept our lives, for our lives, as they have been, have shaped our present identity. With different people and circumstances, we would be different persons. In acceptance, we may achieve fulfillment and integrity. With faith and trust in the Spirit, we may then pray with Simeon,

> Almighty God, you can let your
> servant die in peace,
> just as you promised;

because I have seen the salvation
   which you have prepared for
      all of us to see,
a light to guide us,
   your frail elders, and the glory
      of all people.

2:41-50 / The Boy Jesus in the Temple

While John the Baptist's "hidden life" was in the desert, Jesus' hidden life was in Nazareth. When he was twelve, he left Nazareth with Mary and Joseph to go up to Jerusalem for the Passover. We observe the worry of Mary and Joseph occasioned by the absence of the boy Jesus from the caravan when they were returning to Nazareth. When Jesus, who had remained in the Temple, reminded Mary and Joseph that he must be in his Father's house, Mary and Joseph did not understand and worried about what Jesus meant.

When those of us who are parents saw our children become adults and leave home, we no doubt were relieved that we no longer needed worry about them. Now we may find that we do worry—when a child has lost a job of many years, or when a child's marriage has dissolved, or when other problems arise. That Mary and Joseph worried about Jesus may console us who worry, sometimes because we do not understand our children now that they are adults. Just as Mary "treasured all these things in her heart" (v 51), we might listen to and learn from our children. The worry of Mary and Joseph may also console us when we worry about our grandchildren because they may be unhappy with circumstances in their lives.

2:51-52 / *The Hidden Life at Nazareth*

Reflecting that the childhood and most of the adult years of Jesus' life were in obedience and hidden but, nevertheless, were times of growth, may enable those among us who are shut-ins to accept and even cherish a life that is cut off from the mainstream of activity and that is hidden and unknown sometimes even by neighbors. In noting Jesus' growth in wisdom, stature, and favor, we who are shut-ins may be encouraged to learn how to live meaningful lives within hiddenness and how to grow spiritually and psychologically.

Thus, we are free to devote time each day to prayer, scripture reading, other spiritual reading, and spiritual reflection or meditation.

We might prayerfully recall past experiences, people, and decision points in our lives. Reflecting on our past, we might gain understanding of ourselves in relation to God in the present. Utilizing our prayer, spiritual reflection, and review of the past, we might discern how to live in the present and what shape we want our relationships with family, friends, and those about us to take.

Prayerfully we might reflect on our dying. Preparation for dying might include formulating messages we want to relay to loved ones, mending broken relationships, and implementing the practical transactions needed before dying (such as preparing a will). Recording our thoughts and prayers in our journals, which we can re-read from time to time, may enable us to clarify our thinking, to guarantee our remembering, to gain objectivity and perspective, and to live in the presence of our God.

Prelude to Jesus' Public Ministry

LUKE 3

3:1-20 / *The Proclamation of John the Baptist*

The gospels of Mark and of John (after a prologue) begin with the preaching of John the Baptist. Luke's gospel (as does Matthew's) begins with the infancy narrative. In its glorification of the poor and lowly and reversal of established values, Luke's infancy narrative sets the stage for the story of Jesus' ministry. Luke's gospel then continues with the story of John the Baptist. John, as the transitional person between the periods of Israel and of Jesus, announced the coming of Jesus, who would baptize "with the Holy Spirit and fire."

That John preached repentance to the people of his time as a means of preparing for the coming of Jesus may comfort us who may be laden with guilt just at the time we are preparing for Jesus' coming in death. John's very preaching means that forgiveness is assured to us who repent.

In addition to preaching repentance, John answered the question, "What should we do, then?" for three groups who were listening to

him. He responded to the people that they
must share with those in need what is in excess
of their own basic needs, to the tax collectors
that they must exact only the approved taxa-
tion rate, and to the soldiers that they must not
extort fees but be content with their salaries.
John preached justice and charity.

As we plan our older years, we would do
well to heed John's instruction to prepare spiritually for the coming of Jesus to us through
repentance and through accepting forgiveness.
We might prepare materially through exercising just and charitable stewardship. Those of
us with possessions in excess of our needs
might share what we can with the very needy.
We might take care in justice to do our fair part
in supporting government, community pro-
jects, church, and charities.

3:21-38 / Jesus' Baptism

The baptism of Jesus, which in Luke in-
augurates Jesus' Galilean ministry, may have
been an initiation rite into his new role, under-
taken through the guidance of the Spirit, his
earlier role having been that of a local carpenter. Jesus was about thirty years old when the
Spirit descended on him while he was praying,

when a voice from heaven proclaimed Jesus Son, and when he began his new role. Yet the life expectancy during the time of Jesus was twenty-five years.

We older persons may wonder whether Jesus, as he began his public life, was like the thirty year old of today, or whether he may have reached the human level of maturity of today's older person. Reflecting that Jesus may have been more mature than the young Jesus we usually depict and that he left the role of earlier years to accept a drastically different role may help those of us who have found adjusting to a new retirement role difficult. Jesus left his home, the carpenter shop, his mother and friends in Nazareth to begin the work to which the Father had called him—a work which thrust him into the public milieu. The adjustment must have been great.

Retirement may bring us to a whole new way of living, for which we may not have prepared. Our daily contacts may be with different people. Our time schedules may change drastically. Priorities may be inverted. Whereas household tasks may have been secondary before retirement, after retirement they may be primary and preempt most of our time and attention. A major adjustment is required of us.

Realizing that Jesus made such an adjustment may strengthen us and help us accept difficulty in adjusting to the changes at turning points in our lives.

LUKE 4

4:1-13 / *The Temptation of Jesus*

"Full of the Holy Spirit," Jesus left the scene and occasion of his baptism by John "and was led by the Spirit in the wilderness, where for forty days he was tempted by the devil." As we leave the active roles of younger years for less active roles and more time for ourselves, we may recognize the Spirit in our situations, drawing us to prayer and perhaps to retreat (in the desert). For some of us, the desert may be a nursing home, where we are isolated from the companionship of family and friends and from society.

In Luke's account, the devil first tempted Jesus to change a stone into a loaf. Jesus countered, "One does not live by bread alone" (see Dt 8:3). When our small fixed income has been depleted because of inflation and we are faced with a crisis, such as the serious illness of a spouse and no money for medications, we may

24

be tempted in desperation to violate our deepest values and to act on the principle that "bread alone" is important. Relying on Jesus, who resisted such a temptation, we must seek a way to say "No" and to be true to our values. The way may be that of humbly seeking help from family, friends, our church, or a charitable agency. (A society that so tempts us is indeed a devil.)

Jesus rejected the devil's second temptation, which was to worship the devil in order to acquire the power and glory of possessing kingdoms. For those of us who are frail, the values that we may need to forego in favor of valuing God above all (see Dt 6:13) may be such "ordinary" values as living independently in our own home, determining our own schedules, or even deciding when and what we are going to eat. The threat of losing these ordinary values or the reality of having lost them may result in our being obsessive regarding them.

We might rather do homage to God and serve God alone by accepting our stage of God-given life, with its limits and with its possibilities and its nearness to our eternal goal with God. We might do homage and serve God by living our last stage of life in Jesus' Way.

For those of us who are anxious regarding financing years of frailty, placing need for economic security in Jesus' perspective does not imply that we ought to abandon all concern and await God's action to take care of needs. We are responsible to God for our lives, for planning and making the decisions that enable us to meet our needs, present and future. Jesus countered the final climactic temptation that, if he be the Son of God, he should risk his life by throwing himself down from the parapet of the Temple in Jerusalem: "Do not put the LORD your God to the test" (Dt 6:16).

Jesus' Exit from the Desert

The events preceding and accompanying Jesus' birth presaged his mission as Son of God. His hidden life in Nazareth and the forty-day retreat to the desert prepared him for his mission. Now, at the end of his retreat, the devil left him, and "filled with the power of the Spirit," he, the Son of God, went to Galilee to begin his mission.

As we enter the Galilee of our later years, we bring with us all that influenced us in the past. Perhaps we pause and reflect back on our youth in thought and prayer. And we ask ourselves, "Just how did our parents and others near us, as well as our surroundings, affect us?"

Jesus' retreat into the desert may have been his immediate preparation for his mission. How are we preparing for our still older years and our mission during these years?

Chapter Two

Jesus' Galilean Ministry

The Passion narratives are the oldest sections of the gospels. Drawing on preached accounts of the ministry of Jesus, including sayings, parables, and miracles, the evangelists next wrote accounts of Jesus' ministry, which they arranged in logical, rather than chronological, order. The synoptics (Matthew, Mark, and Luke) did not write of a Judean ministry, as did John, and Luke omitted any journeys outside of Galilee until the journey to Jerusalem.

4:14-30 / Jesus at Nazareth

As we reflectively walk with Jesus, who concluded his forty-day retreat in the desert and began his active ministry with the people of his time, we might recall the beginnings of new roles at key points in our adult lives. We might reflect on the ways in which God walked with us as we grew.

After leaving the desert, Jesus, according to Luke, returned to Galilee, "filled with the power of the Spirit." In Nazareth Jesus went into the synagogue, as was his custom. He read Isaiah 61:1,2 and then proclaimed, "Today this scripture has been fulfilled."

The Spirit, Jesus reads, sent Jesus to bring good news to the poor. Many of us are really poor, particularly those who have been ill for many years or who have depleted resources by caring for sick spouses. We may find comfort and courage in Jesus' mission to bring good news to the poor.

Captive within our homes, or perhaps bound to beds or wheelchairs, the frail among us may rejoice in Jesus' mission to proclaim release to captives, for faith and prayer may lead us to find an inner freedom in union with Jesus.

Jesus came to bring sight to the blind. When anxious about our present or future situations, we may find new sight in the understandings we attain when reflecting on our past, understandings that enable us to accept our lives, find meaning in life, achieve integrity, and bring troubling events to resolution, sometimes through reconciliation with friends or family members from whom we have been alienated. New sight may indicate to those of us who are frail how to live more deeply and fully within the limitations imposed by weakness, immobility, and chronic illness, and especially how to live spiritually in ever-deepening union with Jesus.

Jesus came "to let the oppressed go free." What a consolation this phrase is to the anxious among us who may foresee oppressive situations! Those on Supplemental Security Income may face the frequent threat of reduction or loss of income. Some of us may have family members who, frightened by our increasing frailty, are placing us in nursing homes without consulting us and when institutionalization is not necessary.

The phrase is consoling to the dying ninety-five year olds among us who are plagued by tubes connecting them to sophisticated life-support systems—despite a carefully documented "living will" authorizing the removal of extraordinary supports. Even under these kinds of circumstances, they can rely on Jesus to set them free by his very presence now and, after death, in eternal life. In life after death, their status will be reversed: they shall be truly free.

When reflecting on our lives, we may tend to look at the past and the present in terms of achievements, successes, and usefulness to others—a tendency which may result in feelings of guilt and despair because of past failures and present limitations to achieving and to rendering service. However, the loving concern of Jesus for the poor, captives, blind, and downtrodden attests dramatically to our dignity on the basis of our existence alone.

"Doubtless you will quote to me this proverb, 'Doctor, cure yourself,' and tell me, 'Do here also in your hometown the things that we have heard you did at Capernaum'." Jesus refused to perform wonders for his hometown people in Nazareth, boldly stated that no prophet is accepted in his hometown, and then cited instances where the prophets Elijah and Elisha favored non-Israelites. The people would have thrown him over a cliff, but he eluded them and went his way.

For whatever reasons, persons closest to those of us who are frail may not be the ones best able to respond to our needs. Realizing this phenomenon, instead of castigating family or friends for failing in their "duty," we might accept help from others such as social agencies and parish groups. At the same time, we might cultivate good relationships with family and friends.

4:31-37 / Jesus Teaches in Capernaum and Cures a Man with an Unclean Spirit

How distressing it must be to the older Alzheimer patients among us who realize at times of lucidity that they are often mentally ill and exhibit personalities different from their normal personalities, and that they cause prob-lems for caregivers because of their confusion. That Jesus freed the man of the unclean spirit by his word offers hope that somehow Jesus might respond to those who suffer from Alzhe-imer's Disease. His love for them and their belief and trust in this love may develop in them a generalized sense of well being. This feeling may be akin to the general sense of well being experienced by the infant who is loved and fondled but who is incapable of understanding his/her situation. The feeling of well being stemming from their trust in Jesus' love might free them to live fully during times of lucidity.

4:38-44 / A Number of Cures

The realization that many friends and loved ones and many in our own generation are chronically and/or acutely ill may cause despondency, especially in those of us who are anxious about future frailty. Jesus' response to, and cures of, groups of sick persons may be reassuring, for we know that Jesus will respond to us when we are sick in ways best for each of us.

There are, of course, other possible reflections regarding the stories of Jesus' cures. We may wonder why we or loved ones are not cured. Discouragement with declining, rather than improving, physical conditions and disillusionment from receiving no apparent answers to prayers might result in embitterment. Despite Jesus' compassionate, loving approach to the sick and other marginal persons, we, when distressed because of continually failing health, may agonize over whether lack of faith or some other personal failings may have been the reasons we, or even loved ones, have not been cured.

However, reflection that consistently emphasizes Jesus' basic attitudes (especially love and compassion) and his mission (Lk 4:18) would assure us that Jesus would not withhold cures because of our faults or disposition. Moreover, we may recognize that just as Jesus did not intervene in the course of events that resulted in his own suffering and death, so he normally will not intervene to reverse the course of an illness. Rather, with compassion for us and/or loved ones, he will be present to strengthen, console, and enlighten.

LUKE 5

5:1-11 / Jesus Calls the First Disciples

After preaching from Simon's boat, Jesus directed Simon to let down his nets. When Peter obeyed and saw the bulging nets, he fell at Jesus' knees, "Go away from me, Lord, for I am a sinful man." Despite Peter's confession to sinfulness, Jesus invited Peter to "catch people." Jesus knew and loved Peter. Jesus knew and loved us always—throughout our long lives. He knows and loves us as persons with our peculiar personality traits, environments, and experiences, with our sinfulness. We may indeed feel cherished, as was Peter.

The catch of fish by Peter and his partners, James and John, even though a miracle, indicated that these three men were successful in their work as fishermen. Yet, when Jesus told Peter that from that time he would catch people, Peter, with James and John, left everything and followed Jesus.

Like the first disciples, we may follow Jesus in the special vocation of the older years. Leaving the activities and life styles of younger years and bringing knowledge and experience from the past, we may enter the last stage of life, the last stage of spiritual life on earth. We, hitherto anxious about the future, might discern how Jesus is calling us to a new role of catching people. Realizing the "generative" responsibility that we, as elders, have to society, we might search for a way to share with others the wisdom we may have gained over the years, particularly our learnings regarding Jesus' Way and living that Way. With abandon, we might discern and activate our new roles as

Jesus' followers and, therefore, as persons who are sensitive and reach out to those in need.

5:12-16 / *Jesus Cleanses a Leper*

Jesus' cure of the leper attests to Jesus' commitment to his mission statement (Lk 4:18). Lepers were not only sick, they were social outcasts. Mosaic Law prohibited contact with them. Under Mosaic Law, having certain skin diseases made a person ritually impure and required the person to remain apart from ritually clean members of the community. Yet Jesus "stretched out his hand," touched the leper, and affirmed that, of course, he wanted to cure the leper. The man was cured and thereby freed to be with other persons.

Having lived our younger years during the Great Depression, we may have internalized the value of bodily beauty as a result of viewing beautiful movie stars in films that were our recreation (and perhaps our fantasies). Consequently, we may be overly conscious of the changes in our physical appearance. Moreover, those of us who are frail may be sensitive to a fragile, weak image and may hope that visitors will not notice bed sores, if sores have developed. We may perceive friends, relatives, and caretakers as avoiding us because of the unattractive picture we present.

We know, however, that Jesus does not avoid us but rather seeks us with love and compassion. Through Jesus' love, we become persons of special dignity and worth; we may feel free, therefore, of concern regarding our physical appearance.

5:17-26 / Jesus Heals a Paralytic

When reflecting on the cure of the paralyzed man, which caused the people to be astounded and to praise God, we may feel especially touched by Jesus' initial approach, "Friend, your sins are forgiven you." Jesus, the Son of Man, knew unerringly, we might think, that what the paralytic needed most was forgiveness and freedom from the guilt that plagued him.

In reviewing our lives, we may find ourselves guilt-ridden because we have omitted important deeds and/or committed deeds we consider wrong. We may hunger for freedom from guilt in the assurance that past sins are forgiven. Reflecting on this passage, we may well be assured that Jesus does forgive us. With the comfort of Jesus' forgiveness and of his concern for us, we may be freed of paralyzing guilt and take up our lives with renewed hope.

5:27-32 / Jesus Eats with Sinners in Levi's House

The tax collector Levi, whom Jesus called to follow, and the tax collectors with whom Jesus ate might have been considered betrayers of the community and, therefore, enemies. Jesus associated with them as friends. While some of the persons whom society of today shuns might be dangerous to us if we befriend them, we know and can trust others—the mentally retarded adult across the hall who was robbed, the neighbor's child who was abused, the refugee who does not know how to shop or travel on the bus. Instead of ignoring them, we might listen to them so that they may feel that we understand and care. Perhaps then we can find a way to help or offer suggestions for where to find help.

Mindful of Jesus' response to outcasts, we can act on behalf of those who might pose a danger to a befriender by opposing legislation that discriminates against them and supporting legislation that helps them. Striving to discern Jesus' Way, we might act on such issues as the death penalty, health care for all, and laws forbidding discrimination against gay persons—even if resulting taxes would reduce our resources.

LUKE 6

6:12-19 / Jesus Chooses the Twelve Apostles

Jesus spent the whole night in prayer to God. When day came, he selected twelve of the disciples, whom he called "apostles." Before this important action, as before each important action, according to Luke, Jesus retreated to pray.

We older persons are approaching the most important event and goal of our lives—eternal life. We may welcome, therefore, the time reduced activities allow us to retreat with Jesus in prayer, while we cherish alone times because they provide the climate for prayer. Through prayer we may grow in the knowledge and love of our God with whom we are and will be for eternity. In prayer we might reflect on our past and then on the present in light of the past.

Cherishing our remaining years, we might live each day as prayerfully and therefore as fully as possible. Every event, our joys, our frustrations, our pains and illnesses, and our decisions might all be incorporated into our prayer and enrich it. Finally, we might prayerfully draw our earthly lives to closure in death that we may live for all eternity in prayerful union with our God.

6:20-26 / The First Sermon—The Beatitudes

When Jesus instructed the disciples in what Luke presents as the Sermon on the Plain, his first instruction, in contrast to what the world considered important, valued as happy those who were poor, who were hungry, or who wept. He promised that they would be rewarded.

Many among us are economically poor. Those of us who are frail older persons may suffer the deprivations of poverty and of hunger because of circumstances, such as not being able to shop and obtain necessities or being totally dependent on a caregiver for all necessities. To the poor Jesus promised the kingdom of God, where the king extends mercy.

The active among us may have committed ourselves to helping a frail parent. At the very time our assistance is needed, we may become ill. In the poverty that is our illness, our frail parent may be the one who helps us. Knowing our poverty, we are assured that the kingdom of God is ours. Instead of yielding to feelings of guilt, we might be gentle with ourselves, as well as with our parent.

We, by virtue of having lived longer, usually have suffered losses more extensively than have younger persons. We have known the death of a spouse, of friends, and, some of us, of children; we have experienced the loss of freedom through physical disabilities; and we have known the losses that change brings. We have many losses for which to weep and grieve.

In suffering, we are in solidarity with Jesus and with our peers. Through suffering, we grow. The very causes of our suffering, Jesus tells us through the disciples, mark us as special in the eyes of God, for God is merciful and will reward us in heaven.

6:27-38 / Love of Enemies

In the second part of the Sermon on the Plain, Jesus says, "Love your enemies." Our enemies, according to Luke's Jesus, are those who hate us, who curse, abuse or strike us, or who take our possessions.

"Love your enemies." Jesus asks what seems like the impossible. For those of us who are frail, enemies might be caregivers, even loved ones, who, frustrated and burned out by continuous personal care of us, may, in their efforts to cope, develop hostility toward us; or our enemies might be the same caregivers whose hostility and frustration result in abuse. We, necessarily focusing on neglect or ill treatment, may not consider prayer for, and love of, enemies. Relying on Jesus, who asks such love and instructs us in this virtue, we may grow in understanding such threatened, frightened, and/or burned-out caregivers and even caregivers who knowingly abuse or neglect us. Eventually through Jesus we may pray for our caregivers and even grow to love them.

6:39-42 / *Integrity*

Jesus said to the crowd, "How can you say to your neighbor, 'Friend, let me take out the speck in your eye,' when you yourself do not see the log in your own eye?" At times we may be like the crowd. While in very difficult situations, those of us who are frail and receive care nevertheless may not be conscious of our own failings when thinking or speaking of neglect and/or abuse from others. We may not realize the obstacles we create for caregivers, or our unreasonable demands, complaining, and negativity. Attention to our own personal failings, understandable though these failings may be, may bring the reward of more fulfilling spiritual lives and may even establish a climate in which caregivers and others might respond with improved care.

LUKE 7

7:1-10 / *Jesus Heals a Centurion's Servant*

With the faith of the Roman officer, we might send word to the compassionate Jesus, asking him to heal us of what is causing death in us and therefore is immobilizing us. We might seek healing from our anxiety, worry, guilt, or depression. In faith we know that even while we request help, Jesus is healing us.

7:11-17 / Jesus Raises
the Widow's Son at Nain

The Lord felt sorry for the widow of Nain because her only son was dead. Commanding her dead son to get up, he gave her son back to her. The people praised God, saying, "A great prophet has risen among us" and "God has looked favorably on his people."

Most of us have experienced deaths of a number of people who have been close to us. As difficult as the deaths of our spouses or of close friends are for many of us, the fact that death is expected for the old usually strengthens us to cope. On the other hand, we do not expect our children to precede us in death and, therefore, find the loss of a child particularly painful. Jesus' tender mercy toward the widow of Nain may assure those of us who have lost children in death of Jesus' loving response and of the restoration of life and hope.

7:18-23 / The Baptist's Question

To the question of John the Baptist's disciples, "Are you the one who is to come...?" Jesus referred to the criteria that he had cited in his mission statement (Lk 4:18). He claimed as identifying characteristics the healing of the blind, lame, lepers, and deaf; the raising of the dead; and preaching to the poor.

We are the lame, the deaf, the lepers in need of healing. In addition to the assurance that Jesus will respond to our needs when we are suffering, we are affirmed by Jesus in our self-worth before God, for Jesus identified himself as the one who frees us when we are suffering and downtrodden. Jesus' statement that the person is happy who takes no offense at Jesus strengthens the affirmation.

In answering John's question, Jesus made a statement regarding the values that motivated him. As we prayerfully reflect on our daily lives, we might ask ourselves, "Are we persons who follow Jesus' values, or should those near us look to someone else?"

If children and young adults can see better how to live, relate with others, and make well-reasoned decisions because we share the wisdom gained from our experiences, those who are blind may see. If those of us who are active go shopping for frail, incapacitated neighbors, the lame may walk through us. If we assist in caring for a sick relative, we may help "cleanse" the person of illness. One deaf to values-oriented living might "hear" the message of Jesus simply by observing our sincere efforts to follow Jesus. Our encouragement and affirmation might bring life to a person who has been lifeless because of discouragement. By our efforts to focus on and live Jesus' values, we might indeed be spreading the good news to those whose poverty is deprivation of the "good life."

7:36-50 / *The Sinful Woman*

Jesus not only received the notorious woman sinner, he also accepted her lavish demonstration of love, wherein she kissed his feet and anointed them with ointment. Her love grew out of forgiveness of her sins. In the parable regarding the creditor and two debtors, Jesus showed why the woman's sins were forgiven and the Pharisee's were not; for, in conclusion, Jesus said to the woman, "Your sins are forgiven....Your faith has saved you; go in peace."

We may be guilt-ridden because of sins, real or imagined. Like the woman who came to Jesus, we might approach Jesus and pour out our love for him. Out of our tender love might emerge our sincere sorrow for our offenses. We may be assured that our sins, like those of the woman, are truly forgiven through Jesus' infinite mercy. Knowing that in forgiving our sins Jesus focuses on our love for him rather than on our transgressions, we may live our end time in peace.

In this incident, Jesus emphasized forgiveness and love, but both Jesus and the repentant woman demonstrate other qualities. A notable quality is Jesus' courage in receiving, forgiving, and affirming a woman of unsavory reputation in the presence of the most respected members of the community. Notable also is the woman's courage; knowing her own reputation, she nevertheless entered a room where religious men were dining, wept openly over Jesus' feet, wiped his feet with her hair, and anointed them. Deeply sorry for her sins, she risked humiliation and even repudiation. She had the courage to express her sorrow and love of Jesus in ways she knew.

Sometimes our welcoming or even speaking to a neighbor, a relative, or someone who approaches us may be frowned on by persons whose esteem we value. Establishing a relationship with the person or offering any kind of assistance might be met with disapproval. Relying on Jesus, we might derive courage from a lifetime of experience and risk losing the respect of friends by relating to persons whom these friends do not accept.

LUKE 8

8:1-3 / The Women Accompanying Jesus

The role of the women who accompanied Jesus may have been one of discipleship. Contrary to the customs of his time, Jesus associated with women, dignified them, and granted them an important role in ministry. He responded to women's needs, raising the son of the widow of Nain (7:11-17); forgiving the sinful woman (7:36-50); and curing Simon's mother-in-law (4:38-39), the hemorrhaging woman (8:43-48), the possessed woman (8:2), and a crippled woman (13:10-17). Jesus spoke of women in the parables of the woman and the lost coin (15:8-10) and of the widow and the judge (18:1-8) and praised the widow who gave an offering (21:1-4). Women were key players in Jesus' life drama: Elizabeth, Mary, and Anna in Luke 1 and 2; Martha and Mary (10:38-42); the women at the crucifixion (23:49,55); and the women as witnesses to the empty tomb (24:10-11,22-23).

In the United States, three-fifths of us older persons over sixty-five are women. When we were in our middle years, we might have been involved in our churches through a few auxiliary services. Today, largely through our efforts and the efforts of our sisters and brothers, the roles of lay persons in the church are under study and are expanding, particularly the roles of women.

Each of us might discern our baptismal call to follow Jesus, just as the women Luke mentions accepted Jesus and welcomed and followed him as he preached the kingdom of God. Those of us who have reared children may become the nurturing ministers to the sick, shut-ins, the imprisoned, the poor, and the homeless. We may be communion ministers and nourish our sisters and brothers with the sacramental life of the church. Others of us may apply our life experiences to the planning ministries of our local churches as members of parish councils, finance committees, liturgy committees, and diocesan groups. Knowing the importance of our ministries in the eyes of Jesus, we might consciously witness to his life and resurrection.

8:22-25 / Jesus Calms a Storm

Because of physical disabilities, poverty, weakness, and their aftermath, our lives may be often turbulent and stormy. Pain may rob us forcibly of peace of heart, so that prayer and reflection are difficult.

In the gospel, Jesus used his power to rebuke the wind and waves and bring calm. Might not Jesus rebuke the storm within our hearts and bring us peace and calm? With him we might learn how to cope with our illnesses and disabilities and how to enter into suffering in such a way that we endure and pass beyond our pain to peaceful union with him. In addition, with the realization that Jesus wills peace for us, we may contact doctors and take other possible steps to secure as much pain-free calm in our lives as we can. Prayer and reflection with Jesus may again be integral to our daily lives.

8:26-39 / Jesus Heals the Gerasene Demoniac

At times we may feel beset by many devils within—the devil of a habit of complaining, the devils of paranoia, of depression, of rigidity, of selfishness, of guilt, of worry, of inaction. Jesus took pity on the man possessed with many devils and drove the devils from him.

We, then, may trust that Jesus will be concerned about us and take pity on us. He will respond to our openness and our request to be freed of the devils of unwanted personal characteristics. With our willingness and cooperation, he will help us break habits that enslave us. Having been freed, we may then concentrate our energies in more positive directions— on prayer, on our spiritual development, and on our ministry.

8:40-42,49-56 / Jesus Raises Jairus' Daughter to Life

Longevity has resulted in the phenomenon of some of our children being older persons themselves. As a result, we may worry about adult children who are ill or who are experiencing other problems in their aging process.

Knowing that Jesus responded to Jairus' faith, we may feel free to bring our worries to Jesus. With faith we may ask that he be with our adult older children in their needs. Just as he brought Jairus' daughter to life, he will strengthen our children to cope with their illnesses and problems and enable them to live more fully.

Jesus responded to Jairus, who was so distraught by the serious illness of his daughter that, although president of the synagogue, he knelt before Jesus. When Jairus received word that his daughter had died, Jesus immediately reassured him that, if he had faith, she would be saved. At the home of Jairus, Jesus brought the child back to life. Jesus restored a girl to life, and he did so by taking her hand and speaking to her—in a society that valued boys and especially the only (or oldest) son.

Throughout this incident, Jesus evidenced the respect he accorded all persons, including those whom others looked down on. We, who have encountered many different persons in our long lives, might ask ourselves whether we respect all we meet, including the odd neighbor, the gay young man, and others whom our society may shun. We might ask what our response would be if our neighbor, the young man, or these others needed help.

8:43-48 / Jesus Cures
the Woman with a Hemorrhage

Those of us who have suffered many years from such disabilities as arthritis, angina pectoris, or osteoporosis may feel empathy for the woman who suffered twelve years from a hemorrhage. We may rejoice that Jesus responded instantly to a woman, to a woman who touched him even while she was hemorrhaging. (Under Jewish Law, a man who contacted a hemorrhaging woman became ritually contaminated.)

With faith and hope, we may simply "touch" Jesus in awareness that Jesus cares about us, just as he cared about the woman. When those of us who are frail must concentrate on each action and decision of each day because of memory loss and physical disabilities, we may touch Jesus. When we have difficulty finding meaning in daily living and integrating our lives as we draw close to death, we may touch Jesus. We touch Jesus with faith that Jesus will heal and bring our fragmented lives into wholeness.

LUKE 9

9:1-6 / Mission of the Twelve

Jesus has sent us to proclaim his kingdom and to heal—some of us directly as preachers, all of us indirectly through our lives. As we strive to live Jesus' Way, we might keep in mind those around us, knowing that others, like us, learn by simply observing persons near them. We might share with others the Christian-based thinking we have developed over the years, regarding the important issues concerning ourselves, those near us, and society in general, even while we encourage these same others to share their thinking with us.

Always we might maintain an attitude of hospitality toward others, while accepting their hospitality toward us. In caring, honest dialogue and hospitality, we may further the development of Christian community, the kingdom of God, and enable Jesus' healing influence to touch the often fragmented lives of those near us.

"Take nothing for your journey," Jesus instructed the twelve when he sent them to preach the kingdom of God and to heal. Jesus' instruction may assist us, as we continue our journeys through life, to "let go" psychologically of possessions when, because of physical disabilities or frailty, we need to move to smaller living situations or to institutions. His words may assist us to "let go" of family and friends lost in death and of independence as we become more frail. Finally, Jesus calls us to "let go" of life itself as death approaches.

9:10-17 / Miracle of the Loaves

Jesus was hospitable and generous. Moreover, he may have seized the opportunity to manifest himself more fully to the apostles when he gave them the five loaves and two fishes to distribute among the crowd. The ensuing miracle was a climax to Jesus' Galilean ministry.

Diminished energy, chronic pain, and/or depression may render hospitality and generosity particularly difficult for those of us who are frail. Life is ebbing away. We would well seize the opportunity and, within the limits possible for us, extend hospitality and graciousness toward family, friends, or neighbors. Jesus is manifested in the very relating. He is the source of energy for generosity.

9:18-21 / Peter's Profession of Faith

Jesus had been preaching in Galilee for some time, yet when he asked the disciples who people said he was, they told him that people thought he was John the Baptist, Elijah, or a prophet. Even when we explain over and over again who we are in terms of our living situation, as we grow more frail, we may find our children interpreting what we have said. They may say we need to live near or with them, but re-location uproots us from familiar surroundings where we visit with friends and neighbors.

Jesus asked the disciples, "Who do you say that I am?" Peter identified Jesus as "the Messiah of God," perhaps because he heard Jesus on Jesus' own terms. We might patiently elicit from our children their perceptions of us and then listen carefully. Our own thinking may change, or together we may arrive at a conclusion different from ours or theirs.

Jesus asked, "Who do you say that I am?" Each person needs to develop his/her fundamental faith or philosophy. Each Christian prayerfully needs to develop his/her perception of who Jesus is. For those of us who are frail and are approaching death and Jesus, the perception of who Jesus is becomes particularly important. If we, like Peter, can identify our Jesus with some clarity as "Messiah of God," then we can know Jesus. Knowing Jesus, we can develop a loving and intimate relationship with him. Jesus, then, may become the model of the way we should live our frail years, a model that we follow ever more closely as we approach death and eternal life.

9:22 / First Prophecy of the Passion

Just as Jesus foresaw his suffering and death, so we might look ahead to the day when we must make changes because we are suffering from frailty and diminishments as we approach death. Decisions regarding changes, and the changes themselves, are difficult. In union with Jesus, we might take up the cross of unwanted changes and draw strength from Jesus' sufferings.

It was when Peter perceived Jesus as "the Messiah of God" that Jesus revealed that he, the Son of Man, would be rejected by the Jewish religious leaders, suffer, be put to death, and then be raised up. It is when we who are frail are approaching Jesus and about to know him clearly through death that we may feel rejected by those most important to us, by family and friends, or by the local parish priest, who, because of diminished numbers of priests, is very busy and does not seem to have time for us.

That Jesus was rejected, suffered, and died because of who he was may strengthen us when we are ignored because we are older persons. But Jesus' foreseeing his resurrection may remind us that resurrection and eternal life are also our destiny.

9:23-27 / Conditions for Following Christ

Jesus stated as conditions for following him as a disciple renunciation of self and the daily suffering of the cross, as well as not being ashamed of him and his Way. He did not see shame in suffering, no matter how demeaning the suffering might be in the eyes of many. Rather, he considered shameful the person who is ashamed of him and his teaching.

Those among us who are frail, then, need not be ashamed because we may suffer neglect and careless handling by caregivers. Instead of giving in to feelings of shame, having done what is possible to change abusive conditions, we might follow Jesus in daily taking up the cross and in renunciation of self, drawing strength from Jesus.

9:28-36 / The Transfiguration

When Jesus was overshadowed by a cloud, which signified God's presence, the three apostles heard a voice proclaim Jesus his Son and instruct, "Listen to him." This heavenly identification of God's presence in Jesus' word preceded Jesus' journey to Jerusalem (his city of destiny) and his exodus from there. It parallels the heavenly identification of Jesus during his baptism, the identification that inaugurated his Galilean ministry.

Jesus led the three disciples up a mountain in Galilee, where they might behold broad visions and perspectives. Indeed, the disciples witness the transformation of Jesus, and they themselves may have been transformed.

Jesus may be leading us up the mountain of the next, and perhaps last, period of our lives. He may be broadening our vision of what we might do in ministry, so that we might become capable of one-to-one personal service to a frail older person. Like Peter, we may become open to knowing Jesus in a new way and descend the mountain, transformed.

9:46-48 / Who Is the Greatest?

As Jesus was concluding his Galilean ministry, he emphasized his own humble death and he responded to the disciples, "The least among all of you is the greatest."

For many of us, especially the frail, achievements are in the past; material possessions may be gone; our appearance is altered; and, in place of vigor, there is illness, arthritis, and no energy. That Jesus considers the person at his/ her greatest precisely when society sees the person as the least may offer a sense of self-worth to us who may have internalized Jesus' values of powerlessness and unworldliness.

Many of us have retired. We have lost contact with the people with whom we associated when we were working, among them perhaps people judged prestigious by us and our peer workers. In equating our welcoming him with welcoming a little child, Jesus may be teaching us to welcome the "ordinary" people with whom we live and associate and to value them.

The End of the Galilean Ministry

At this point Luke concludes Jesus' Galilean ministry. It had been a ministry to the poor, the lame, the sick, to and with women and tax collectors. Jesus had challenged legalistic interpretations of the Sabbath with healings on that day. He had preached to the people. He had called the apostles and had been transfigured before them. Now he resolutely took the road to Jerusalem.

The End of Our Ministry of Earlier Days

As we review our early adult years, we ask: What was our attitude toward unfortunate people? How did we bring the good news to others, or liberty, or sight, or freedom? Perhaps we are led by reflection on our younger years to consider our attitude today. To whom does the Spirit send us in this time, our older years?

As older persons, we are likely suffering from some forms of poverty, blindness, or oppression. How is Jesus bringing us good news? How is he freeing us?

Chapter Three

Jesus' Journey to Jerusalem

In the next section of his gospel, Luke presents Jesus as goal-oriented, Jesus' goal being Jerusalem and his mission there. In Jerusalem Jesus will fulfill the Law of Moses and the prophets.

The Journey to Jerusalem

9:51-56 / An Inhospitable Samaritan Village

About six months before his death, as the time drew near for him to be taken up, Jesus "resolutely" set out for Jerusalem, where he would die. During the time preceding the Jerusalem journey, he had prophesied twice regarding his suffering and dying. Perhaps he was living this period of his life from a new perspective gained from his facing imminent death. Perhaps this perspective heightened the importance of situations and day-by-day decisions, particularly regarding the mission given him by his Father. He may have treasured each moment, living it more intensely and intentionally. Perhaps, too, he experienced freedom with the realization that his goal in life would be fulfilled. He may have grown into a deeper understanding of himself and of the Father and a stronger determination to be more fully himself in the Father.

The "end time," however long it may be, is a very special time. The frail among us, who are reminded daily that time is culminating, might resolutely set out on our final journey. Accepting whatever energy is available to us, we might cherish each moment and situation. We might take care in our relations with those near us and reach out to persons with whom we may need reconciliation. Reflecting on our past, we may grow to a deeper understanding of ourselves in relation to God. Resolving and integrating our past lives into the present, we may experience the final freedom to be more authentically ourselves—the persons God made us to be.

Jesus was intent on achieving his goal, Jerusalem. For this reason, perhaps, he did not address the refusal of the Samaritans to receive him nor the suggestion of James and John (the Sons of Thunder) that they call down fire from heaven to burn up the Samaritans. As we who are frail focus on our final journey, we may find that some situations no longer concern us, when in the past they always elicited a response from us. Our newly focused perspective frees us to respond only to what achieves our end, eternal life in the new Jerusalem.

9:57-62 / Hardships of Following Jesus

As we who are anxiously regarding our future older years endeavor to follow Jesus, we may learn the relentless detachment that following Jesus entails. We may indeed leave behind homes of our own as we plan for retirement into housing set aside for older persons. In time we may let go psychologically of our loved ones who have died and concentrate our energies on relating to our few remaining relatives and/or friends, who may now be dying and must be left behind. We may know only too well that there is no turning back.

There is no turning back as we follow Jesus. If the three persons in this passage had accepted Jesus' invitation, they would have become his disciples and, perhaps, witnesses of his resurrection. What a privilege they relinquished! We might well ask ourselves whether we are discerning the call that Jesus extends to each of us. His call is to a privileged discipleship in our remaining older years, including our day-by-day living.

For the frail among us, following Jesus in service to others may mean limiting requests for help to what we cannot do for ourselves. Persons who might otherwise expend all their time and energy caring for us might then be free to pursue other kinds of discipleship to which Jesus may be calling them.

Following Jesus' call may mean making ourselves available for listening to troubled relatives and neighbors and for socializing with them. Jesus may be calling us who are more active to minister in a special way to those who are frail, especially the frail who are shut-ins. These lone frail persons may have no close friends or relatives, no persons with whom to carry on significant conversations. While visiting them, we might be sensitive to remarks that indicate a desire to pursue topics important to them. Showing our interest, we might encourage our frail friends to share their thoughts with us. We might deliberately exercise creative listening, which seeks accuracy in hearing the content our friends convey and in "hearing" the accompanying feelings.

Thus, we may enable the frail to understand their own thinking objectively and to arrive at important decisions. Our ministry of listening may enable persons near death to review the past, to find meaning in it, and to achieve integrity in their lives. In a few cases, we may be able to facilitate persons' reconciling themselves with estranged relatives. More often, we may enable the frail to work through guilt feelings or life situations that have troubled them to occasional expressions of sorrow, acceptance of what has been, and closure. We may be ministers who facilitate the persons' preparations for death and eternal life.

LUKE 10

10:25-37 / Parable of the Good Samaritan

The anxious among us may worry about societal world situations. Moreover, we may have experienced a mugging or a cat burglar who took money and left us with a feeling of insecurity. At the same time, we may be sincerely concerned about the homeless, persons with AIDS, those afflicted by the drug problem, our frail elderly and their families, or those who are battered and victimized. How can we be neighbor to these persons?

In the parable of the Good Samaritan, Jesus reinforced the commandment to love our neighbor. He taught love of neighbor modeled on the way God loves. In presenting an extreme example, Jesus demonstrated that love takes pity on the neighbor and extends even to the neighbor who is considered in popular opinion to be as despicable as the Samaritans were to the Jews.

The Samaritan performed simple, neighborly tasks. Our response toward the needy whom we tend to ignore or pass by may be simple. For some of us, response may take the form of supporting others who can help more actively through our encouragement and/or financial support. Others of us may find that we can help the poor or drug abusers through the work we choose and by volunteering. Like the Samaritan we need to be open to the situations that confront us and to different ways of helping. Our openness will affect on-the-spot decisions, how we vote, what we say, and it will therefore contribute to public opinion and the formation of laws. Whatever response we make, it should be offered with the compassion that characterized the Samaritan in the parable.

10:38-42 / Martha and Mary

Mary, who sat at the Lord's feet and listened to him, chose the better part in contrast to Martha, who was "distracted by her many tasks." Some of us older persons may have developed overly busy lives, with little or no time for prayer. We might well examine our daily routines and make the necessary adjustments for time and a quiet place to sit with the Lord. For those of us whose working children expect long hours in babysitting and/or housekeeping from us, listening at Jesus' feet may at times suggest limiting or foregoing these tasks.

For others of us whose parents may be living but failing in health, listening at Jesus' feet may be hearing Jesus in the voice and needs of our parents. We cannot hear Jesus unless we pause to sit at his feet and listen. We might hear again the message regarding his compassionate responses to individual people who were in need and hurting. Perhaps at this time in our lives, we might hear the call to minister one-to-one in a reflective, hidden stance.

Just as in reflection and in dialogue with others we found ways to engage in active parish ministry, perhaps as communion ministers to shut-ins, so in listening to Jesus, we may find ways now to be "care-givers," ways that are ministerial to our parents and life-giving to us. Jesus might be showing us "the better part."

The frail among us who may feel guilty about not serving Jesus by serving others may rejoice in our forced role of passivity and welcome the opportunity to sit at the Lord's feet and listen. As in Psalm 77:4-6, we may pray,

> You keep my eyelids from
>   closing;
> I am so troubled that I cannot
>   speak.

I consider the days of old,
   and remember the years of
     long ago.
I commune with my heart in the
     night;
   I meditate and search my spirit.

LUKE 11

11:1-4 / The Lord's Prayer

As we reflect carefully on the model prayer Jesus taught us, we realize that prayer is worship of God. Yet we marvel that Jesus chose the intimate, loving appellation "Father" to designate the God we worship. We pray that the Father may reign in our hearts and in the hearts of all. The Father's values, then, will be our values, the values taught by Jesus. We remind our provident Father of our daily needs. Acknowledging, naming as sins, and renouncing our failures to live the Father's values, we confidently ask for forgiveness, even as we strive to forgive those who have offended us. Finally, with hope we seek preservation from trials too great for us.

With new-found time at our disposal, the frail among us who had been very active and now have little energy might appreciate the manner of praying taught by Jesus and pray in our own words,

> Father, may we revere You.
> May You reign in our hearts.
> Grant that our daily needs be fulfilled.
> Forgive us our sins,
> for, with Your help,
>> we strive to forgive those
>> who do not perform
>> their duty toward us.
> And do not allow us trials beyond our
> endurance.

11:14-20 / Jesus and Beelzebub

In casting out the devil from a dumb man, Jesus presented a sign for the poor, a sign different from that his opponents wanted. In effect, he was telling his opponents that their thinking was not logical when they asserted that he cast out devils through Beelzebub.

We may be startled by the new ways of following Jesus described in the diocesan newspaper or church bulletin, such as protests at nuclear sites and campaigns regarding legislation that affects the poor. We may then criticize negatively Christians involved in such "untraditional" activities. Reflection on the illogical criticism of Jesus by his opponents may indicate to us who subscribe to Jesus' Way of peace and concern for the poor that, in criticizing those promoting peace and justice, our thinking is illogical. We may instead replace negative criticism with support, for "Whoever is not with me is against me" (v 23).

LUKE 12

12:13-21 / On Hoarding Possessions

In relating the parable of the rich fool, Jesus taught that "life does not consist in the abundance of possessions" (v 15). Fear of insecurity or of the depletion of resources because of a long stay in a convalescent hospital may motivate some of us who are anxious to hoard possessions far beyond what we need, to the neglect of the just needs of others. Reflection on Jesus' teaching may encourage us to save prudently what is needed and to give generously to others, thereby making ourselves "rich toward God."

We may ask ourselves, however, the meaning of being rich before God. Certainly, they are rich who have become as fully as possible the persons God made them to be. For the riches we bring to God are the developed riches God placed in us as incipient capacities, riches which we were free to develop or to allow to remain dormant.

With new-found leisure, those of us who have retired may have discovered abilities that we did not know were within us. We are privileged to develop these talents, to share them with others, and, in so rounding out our personalities, to become more fully the persons potentially present in us at creation. Then we may stand before God, truly rich.

12:35-40 / On Being Ready for the Master's Return

Church personnel, hospice groups, psychologists, hospital chaplains, and others have made themselves available to assist persons who are dying. It would seem that Jesus sanctioned and proposed careful preparation for death when he called for readiness for the return of the master, for the coming of the Son of Man; in fact, he declared the prepared person happy. The availability of persons to assist with dying is a new concept to most of us. When we are frail, we might consider this kind of help as we prepare for death.

At all times and with ever-new readiness, we must be ready for Jesus' coming, for he is always coming and always with us. Just as the loving spouse greets, welcomes, and receives the loved one anew with every encounter, so we want to greet Jesus and welcome and receive him over and over. We want our relationship with him to be ever new. Those of us who are retired want to use our time and opportunity to renew our relationship with Jesus many times a day.

12:49-50 / Jesus and His Passion

Jesus, who gave himself totally to fulfilling the Father's mission for him, was impatient for this mission to emblaze the entire world. Goal-oriented, he was impatient also for his final baptism in his Passion and death. We who profess to follow Jesus might live according to his teachings zealously and "publicly." In sharing with others the gospel values according to which we live, we may set our small part of the world on fire.

The frail among us are approaching a baptism we might still receive, our suffering before death. We might pray in union with Jesus, who suffered. Our suffering may simply take the form of fearing the unknown and of the stark aloneness of dying. Like Jesus, we, while fearful, may be distressed by the very waiting for death, particularly if we are unaccountably lingering or being kept alive by extraordinary life supports. We might pray and strive for the grace to confront suffering and actively live it.

LUKE 13

13:10-17 / Jesus Heals a Crippled Woman on the Sabbath

The disabled woman, feeling his gentle touch, knew that Jesus cared personally about her in her bondage. When Jesus saw the woman, he voluntarily healed her. Criticized for healing on the Sabbath, Jesus responded, "...[O]ught not this woman, a daughter of Abraham whom Satan bound for eighteen long years, be set free from this bondage on the sabbath day?" Jesus' cures freed ailing persons of illnesses that held them in bondage; freedom of the person was an important value to Jesus. In fact, he was so concerned for the person's freedom and life, that he disregarded ritual impurity and laid hands on a sick woman.

The disabled among us, like the people of Jesus' time, may be overjoyed by the fact that Jesus, without prompting or a request for help, called the woman to him and freed her by healing her. Might not Jesus, then, draw to himself those of us who are physically or psychologically disabled and effect the kind of healing most needed by us?

Might not Jesus effect also the freedom most needed? For the frail among us who find ordinary personal tasks and household chores horrendously difficult and energy-consuming, the freedom to be ourselves with Jesus may consist in accepting the unfreedom of institutional care. Freed thereby from the laborious difficulty of these ordinary tasks, we may have time and energy to explore self, to reflect on the past, and to pray in union with Jesus.

13:34-35 / Jerusalem Admonished

Luke portrays Jesus as seeing his arrival in Jerusalem as his goal. In Luke's perception,

Jerusalem was the place of revelations, the link with the beginning church. It was the holy place to Jesus and his people, because the Temple was there. Yet, the leaders of its people had killed the prophets. As with his own suffering and death, Jesus, who loved the holy city, understood and had compassion on the people. Like a hen, he would gather them under his wings.

We, who have been privileged to know Jesus and his church, by that very fact stand in our world's holy place. At times our leaders and we have made serious mistakes, and we as church have participated in horrendous scandals, with responsibility even for killing. Jesus in forgiving still loves his holy church and understands and has compassion for us, its people.

He has compassion for us who are older, as we strive to live his way in our unique roles in the church, even with our mistakes. We might be reassured that, now and when we are dying, Jesus will draw us near him under his tender protection, "as a hen gathers her brood under her wings." "Blessed is the one who comes in the name of the Lord!"

LUKE 14

14:7-11 / On Choosing Places at Table

To those who would choose the highest positions for themselves, Jesus taught the counter-cultural value of humility in choosing the lowest positions. Each of us might well ask as we approach the end of life,

- What are my values?

- How important to me is the good opinion of society in general or of those around me?

- Might I not accept the humble position others assign me because of my age and disabilities, while not approving their attitude, knowing that God exalts me?

As we retire from the work with which we may have identified for many years, we might encourage and assist younger persons to replace us and to seek other responsible positions. Where we can, we might humbly offer to share insights and skills we have gained over the years. In our extended family circles, too, we might relinquish our leadership positions to younger family members. As we facilitate

positions of honor for the young, our own position of honor may be the background seat
from which we may savor the success of the
young, which we in some ways enabled.

14:12-14 / On Choosing Guests to Invite

Instead of yearning for the company of
those whose friendship we may see as prestigious, advantageous, or simply desirable, we
might cherish the friendship of those who respond to us. Those who respond may be other
older persons in similar situations or in less
favorable circumstances than ours: "the poor,
the crippled, the lame, the blind," the persons
whom Jesus recommended we invite to a meal
and to whom he promised the kingdom of God
(Lk 6:20).

14:25-27 / The Cost of Discipleship

To be Jesus' disciples, we must follow him
and espouse his values totally and unremit-
tingly. Whatever violates or compromises
these values must, for that reason, be rejected
and ignored. This stance in itself is hard and
constitutes our cross.

To be Jesus' disciples, we must be so true to
his Way that at times we must live and act

contrary to our own natures and our deepest, most valid desires. Some of us must perforce endure ongoing illness and excruciating pain. We must take up and carry our cross.

For those of us who are dying, perhaps the renunciation for which Jesus calls is a willingness to give up family and friends who have died or moved away. Eventually, Jesus calls for the willing renunciation of self in death. The renunciation may be painful and may be part of the cross we bear in order to follow Jesus.

LUKE 15

15:1-10 / The Lost Sheep

The fifteenth chapter of Luke emphasizes God's mercy toward sinners and God's joy when one sinner repents. In response to the criticism of the scribes and Pharisees that he welcomed sinners and ate with them, Jesus asked who would not leave ninety-nine sheep in the wilderness and seek the one lost sheep. Thus Jesus emphasized the value and dignity of each person before God, even when the person is sinning.

We might ask ourselves whether we truly believe in God's tender, all-forgiving love. Our prayer might be for faith and the ability to respond, willingly accepting God's forgiveness of us who are sinners. Upon being carried back to the fold, we might rejoice and integrate ourselves into our local communities of faith.

We anxious ones, who are habitually in doubt concerning our own "righteousness" before Jesus and who are therefore worried, may be reassured by Jesus' parable. The Good Shepherd, Jesus, will seek us sinners and bring us back on his shoulders to the fold, back to following him. Following Jesus the Shepherd, we might in turn strive to forgive those closest to us who annoy us, as well as persons who have been seriously unjust to us.

15:11-24 / The Prodigal Son

So insistent was Jesus regarding God's openness to receive the repentant sinner that he reinforced this theme with another parable, that of the prodigal son. The parable is really about the loving father, who is a figure of God. An earthly father might consider his son as separated from him (as though the son were dead) when the son demanded his inheritance and left home. The father in the parable (God) forgives and looks for reconciliation, even before the son determines to ask forgiveness. Not only does the father forgive and reconcile himself with the son when the son asks pardon, but the father even rejoices in the son's return and calls in others to celebrate with them.

We, having reviewed the past and considered ourselves in the present, may be overwhelmed with guilt and sorrow. We are assured forgiveness, however, even if our repentance occurs near the end of life. Moreover, the Father, like the father of the prodigal son, does not view us with the eye of judgment but sees us through the eyes of love. He continually waits and watches for our return. When we return, the Father is "moved with pity" and focuses on celebration and not on retribution. With confidence, then, we may rejoice in forgiveness and reconciliation with the Father.

15:25-32 / The Dutiful Son

Again Jesus corrected the Pharisees' and scribes', as well as our own, perception of God in relation to sinners. Rather than relating to us as slaves or employees, God, as Father, relates to us as children whom He loves infinitely and constantly. God's love does not depend on our goodness or the performance of our duties.

Moreover, just as the father in the parable assumes that the older son will adopt the father's perspective toward the younger son, so God expects us to recognize others as God's children and our brothers and sisters. God's expectation is that we, like God, will love others, always be ready to forgive and welcome others, and rejoice at others' reconciliation and good fortune.

When tending to be self-righteous and to castigate those whom we perceive as sinners (sometimes including our own children) we might learn from the attitude of the generous father of the prodigal. Instead of relating to others as strangers and on a judgmental basis, we might relate with them as our brothers and sisters, whom we accept and love, and whom, because of our love, we forgive in advance of any wrong.

LUKE 16

16:1-8 / The Crafty Steward

With this parable and the instructions that follow sporadically in Luke until the story of the Passion, we may reflect on our stewardship before our master, Jesus. The frail among us might well consider these passages in our pre-paring for death.

The steward in Jesus' parable, who is pre-paring himself for the loss of his stewardship, is good to his master's debtors so that he might be welcome in the debtors' homes. His re-source becomes people and not money (for he could have made a profit for himself by adding to the fifty measures of oil and the eighty meas-ures of wheat owed his master).

As we grow older and loved ones and neighbors either die or move away from us, we may realize how precious are the people in our lives—more precious and important than our financial security. We may recall that Jesus preached love of God and neighbor and there-by charged us with responsibility for relating to others in a loving way.

As we reflect on the past, we might consider how we have exercised stewardship through relationships with persons as well as through administering material goods. We might re-flect on our relationships with our children and spouses and with others near us. Our reflection may help us evaluate how we are presently relating to the persons in our lives. While friends and relations are with us, we, who may lose them in death, may want to seize the opportunity sincerely and responsibly to love and serve them.

16:19-31 / The Parable of the Rich Man and Lazarus

The parable of the rich man and Lazarus, which is a reinforcement of Jesus' enigmatic teaching, "Make friends...by means of dishonest wealth" (v 9), depicts God's judgment on a rich man and a poor man, a judgment that reverses the situations of the two persons and that may be very different from the judgment anticipated by the rich man. In desperation, the rich man asks Father Abraham that his brothers be warned through a miraculous intervention.

As we reflect on the past, some of us may realize that we have lived from day to day, with little motivation, planning, or attention to values. Prayer and serious reflection may have been absent. Possibly we expected some intervention in old age that would set all things aright before death. This parable demonstrates the folly of expecting salvation through miraculous intervention.

Instead, we might begin now seriously to repent and to strive to follow Jesus' Way during our remaining days. Hopefully, a lifetime of habitual neglect has not fixed an impassable gulf between careless living and living based on Christian values.

LUKE 17

17:1-4 / Correcting and Forgiving

Those among us who are frail may live in nursing homes. Some of us may experience abuse. Even though we are frail, we have an obligation to correct the abuse, if there is any way we can do so, for our own sake and for the sake of other residents. We are the only ones who know fully the extent of the abuse. At least, we might tell family or trusted friends what has happened so they may help stop the abuse. Perhaps fearful of reprisals on the part of the nursing home staff, we might take courage from Jesus' directive to reprove the one doing wrong.

Jesus' directive to reprove is coupled with the directive to forgive "seven times a day" if we are offended that often and the offending person is sorry. For Jesus, forgiveness is always. On the cross he extended forgiveness, even when those who crucified him did not express sorrow.

As we review our lives, hurts from the past may surface. Childhood recollections may focus on parents who were cruel or heedless or whose well-intentioned guidance was damaging to the growing child's self-image. Knowing the effect of parental influence on our lives, we may find it difficult to forgive and may be further distressed by guilt because of the inability to forgive.

Asking Jesus to be with us, we might patiently recall feelings of hurt during childhood and since and, placing them before Jesus, seek healing from the hurts. Realizing that every thing, situation, and person that we encountered, including what may have been harmful, contributed to who we are today, we might accept and embrace who we are in Jesus. Gradually we may be able to accept and forgive parents who wronged us long ago.

17:11-19 / Jesus Cleanses Ten Lepers

In addition to their physical disability, lepers suffered ostracism from the community because of the danger of ritually contaminating others. When Jesus healed the ten lepers, he also freed them to seek the companionship of others.

All of us, and especially the frail, may have experienced relief from excruciating pain. We may have brought our pain to Jesus. Yet, when relieved of pain and able to relate again with others, we may have forgotten our terrible suffering. Instead, we focused on the troubles of the moment and, like the nine lepers, forgot gratitude for the many blessings and graces that were also present at that moment. We need to remember our suffering and to express our gratitude to God, who loves us and is intimately involved with our lives.

17:20-21 / The Coming of the Kingdom of God

"The kingdom of God is among you," Jesus instructed. Even when those of us who are frail are alone most of the time, we may be consoled by the mystery of the kingdom of God within us and within all sincere believers in a bond that defies the isolation of the shut-in state.

When the more active among us are with family or friends, the kingdom of God is among us. It is among us when we meet with church groups to determine the quality of our ministries or to discern our individual ministries. We bring the kingdom of God to others when we shop, recreate, or travel and extend the little courtesies and respect that brief encounters with others call forth. The kingdom of God is among us especially when we deliberately offer assistance to the needy and suffering. We need not look for the kingdom but rejoice in its presence among us.

17:22-37 / The Day of the Son of Man

Those of us who are frail shut-ins may long for the coming of the Son in death. There may be signs of Jesus' coming in pneumonia, a heart attack, or a stroke, but Jesus eludes us and comes when least expected. Moreover, during this momentous time of readiness for Jesus' coming, we may experience dismay and even shock with the realization that the rest of the world goes on—our own family and friends continue to eat and drink and engage in daily activities.

We may poignantly experience Jesus' predictions that the end may mean severance from others, for "on that night there will be two in one bed; one will be taken and the other left." In the end we must wait alone for the coming of the Son; throughout our lives, we faced each new stage alone, even when family and friends were there. For it was each of us alone who took the step into adulthood, married, professed faithfulness in religious life, or entered the adult employment world. No one else could enter each new passage for us or with us. We felt our aloneness keenly because of the unknown that lay before us—the unknown in our new life stage and the unknown in our capacity or non-capacity to meet new challenges.

It is each of us alone who will die. No one can die for us nor be truly with us in death. No one can tell us what death is like. However, Jesus did tell us—so, therefore, we do know—that the Son will come to us. It is in this knowledge and hope that we take courage and because of this hope that we may even long for death.

LUKE 18

18:1-8 / The Unscrupulous Judge and the Importunate Widow

Jesus urged the disciples to pray always and never lose heart. As a model of such persistence, he told the story of a widow who sought justice from a judge so insistently that the judge finally responded lest the widow wear him out.

How encouraging this lesson may be to the frail among us who are in dire circumstances— experiencing weakness, poverty, aloneness, without anyone to whom to turn. Never losing hope, we may pray to God, the Judge, while striving continually for readiness for death but also for assistance and strength to live until death. God, who hears the needy, will help us.

All of us have the responsibility of seeking our just needs. Often we must ask for our needs from those who control them and we must continue to ask and even insist on our rights. Jesus instructed us to seek our just needs from God, praying continually. Moreover, he assured us that God will see that justice is done for us. How reassuring!

18:9-14 / The Pharisee and the Tax Collector

"God, be merciful to me, a sinner." These words from a tax collector, the most despised of persons among the Jews, are the words Jesus used to exemplify humility in prayer.

The tax collector may have known that he had sinned—in cheating people, in helping the Romans oppress his community, and in other ways. The Pharisee, who was well respected in the community, did not know himself as a sinner and focused on how much better he was than others.

We have sinned. Through reflection on scripture and on Jesus' Way, we may be able to raise our own awareness of our sinfulness. We may then be able to know our sins and to name them, and humbly to ask for forgiveness and the grace to sin no more.

As we reflect on our past lives, sincere humility may enable gratitude for all that has been good, rewarding, and meaningful. Humility may incite expressions of true sorrow for neglect of others, for participation in what has harmed others, and for failure to live Jesus' Way. Humility may result in healing of spirit and reconciliation with God and with others, when this is possible. Sincere humility may enable us finally to be raised up to God in death and resurrection.

18:31-34 / Third Prophecy of the Passion

Jesus predicted his Passion a third time; yet, Luke writes in three different ways that the apostles did not understand. One wonders what Jesus felt about their obtuseness. Might not the fact that no one responded when Jesus spoke of the dire circumstances which would accompany his death have saddened or even depressed him?

Psychologists maintain that depression is common in today's society and that it is especially common among older persons. Moreover, depression may be an appropriate and healthy response to some very trying circumstances.

Those of us who may be anxious regarding future frailty are often anxious precisely because of the suffering frailty may bring. When attempting to discuss the future with family or friends, we may find that they do not understand, as the apostles did not understand Jesus. Perhaps unconsciously they avoid or cannot face the suffering of a loved one or what might be their own future suffering. Perhaps, with the stress of daily living and relationships, family and friends find looking at our futures too much to endure at the moment.

This lack of understanding and unwillingness to hear may depress us, for it means that we ultimately face suffering and death alone, just as Jesus was alone in the end moments. His aloneness and perhaps depression may somehow strengthen us to accept future suffering and to prepare for it in solidarity with him.

18:35-43 / Jesus Heals a Blind Man

The frail among us may find that we are sitting by the side of the way of life, so that we do not receive the information that comes to persons in the mainstream. Just when we may need healing because of chronic or terminal illnesses which have relegated us to the sidelines, we may learn that the health benefits promised older persons are simply not there. With little energy for coping, we may beg for someone to help us see how to cope with illnesses, obtain life necessities, carry on life tasks, and follow Jesus' Way. We may indeed be blinded.

Patiently, like the blind man near Jericho, we might take hold of our lives and bring them to Jesus, asking that he take pity on us so that we may see how to live his Way in our situations. Jesus will respond himself and, hopefully, through others. Hopefully, too, we will recognize Jesus when he comes through others. Thus, we, like the blind man, may praise God and be joined in praise by those who see the good that has happened.

LUKE 19

19:1-10 / Jesus and Zacchaeus

Jesus noticed Zacchaeus, who was a tax collector for the Romans and therefore someone despised by the Jews; he noticed the extraordinary efforts of Zacchaeus to see him. Jesus honored Zacchaeus by inviting himself to stay at Zacchaeus' house. When Zacchaeus frankly told Jesus that he would give half his property to the poor and would pay back fourfold anyone he had cheated, Jesus announced that salvation had come and that Zacchaeus was indeed a son of Abraham. Jesus totally accepted Zacchaeus, for the Son of Man "came to seek out and to save the lost."

Like Zacchaeus, we may be making extraordinary efforts to "see" Jesus and Jesus' Way. We may be striving to live simply as Jesus did and to provide responsibly for our frail years. At the same time, we may be struggling with how we might respond to the poor and needy, for we, like Zacchaeus, know that Jesus reached out to the poor. We note that Jesus affirmed Zacchaeus' efforts to be just to the poor when he honored Zacchaeus with the appellation "son of Abraham." Jesus will respond to our efforts, totally accept us, and be with us and strengthen us to develop in his Way, for Jesus has been seeking us during all of our lives in order to save us.

19:11-14 / Parable of the Pounds

As Jesus was about to reach the goal of his journey, Jerusalem, he spoke of a king who was rejected by the people. Thus Jesus foreshadowed his own fate in Jerusalem, his rejection as king by his own people.

Having matured beyond our so-called middle years, we are approaching the goal of our life's journey: death and eternal life. We may look back on the span of our adult years and reminisce—recalling what elicited joy and what brought sorrow, when we were affirmed and when rejected. With a renewed sense of wholeness and yet fragmentation in our lives, with the recognition of threads, patterns, and influences as well as disruptions and crises, we might approach anew our last years and enter with Jesus into our Jerusalem.

We might ask ourselves about teachings Jesus left us during his journey to Jerusalem. There is his instruction on prayer and his example. When have we prayed, and in what way? How has our prayer life changed over the years? Did it develop as we developed? Is prayer now guiding us in our older years? How might prayerful discernment of God's call to us in these years enable us to live Jesus' Way more fully?

Chapter Four

Jesus' Jerusalem Ministry

19:28-40 / The Messiah Enters Jerusalem

As Jesus approached Jerusalem, the geographic goal of his journey and of his life on earth, he eagerly went on ahead. To mark his entrance into the city of his goal, he chose to descend from the Mount of Olives, riding into the city on a colt, and to be acclaimed as king by his disciples. The celebration was memorable and beautiful in its simplicity. In Jerusalem Jesus would achieve his goal: suffering, death, resurrection, and ascension.

The frail among us older persons, like Jesus, have entered the Jerusalem of our lives and are approaching our goal: suffering, death, and resurrection. We might celebrate the important passage into the place of our goal with Jesus. Joyfully we might welcome and proclaim anew Jesus as king of our final years, as the one with whom we shall find peace and glory in heaven.

19:45-48 / Jesus in the Temple

Jesus' goal in journeying to Jerusalem was, in Luke's presentation, a goal of being acclaimed as king and therefore also a goal of journeying to the Temple. An assertive Jesus entered the Temple, a Jesus different from the meek and peaceful Jesus of the earlier days of his ministry. In cleansing the Temple, Jesus, acting as prophet, prepared it and then occupied it as his own.

As we grow older, we may find ourselves better able to address wrongs than when we were younger. We may be less afraid and less concerned about what others think of us. Keeping before us our value of justice, just as Jesus pursued his goal, we might assertively address some of the blatant injustices in our society. We might even join with others who are addressing such issues as nuclear disarmament, national health care, and just peace throughout the world.

We might take care to include other appropriate groups of people in our advocacy which addresses needed benefits for the elderly. Thus, in seeking cost-of-living adjustments in Supplemental Security Income, we might also join those seeking adjustments in Aid for Families with Dependent Children.

We as older persons can change and grow. In our efforts toward the elder task of integrating our personalities, we might reflect on potentials within us that have not been developed, on how we might free those qualities to emerge, on how we might develop them, and on how these qualities might serve ourselves and others.

LUKE 20

20:9-19 / Parable of the Wicked Tenants

In the Hebrew Bible, the chosen people are frequently considered God's vineyard, with their leaders as caretakers of the vineyard. But the people treated their leaders, the prophets, shamefully. When God sent the Son, the Son was put to death outside the vineyard.

In telling this parable, Jesus was no doubt referring to the history of his people and to the fact that he himself would be slain outside the walls of Jerusalem. Jesus spoke hard words to his own people: he will "give the vineyard to others." "The stone that the builders rejected has become the cornerstone" (Ps 118:22).

We, as tenants in God's vineyard, might well ask ourselves how we are carrying out our responsibilities. In carrying out our responsibilities, we may at times need to speak the truth out of our experience, to speak hard words to our families or members of our church. These words, like Jesus' words, may be rejected. It may have been necessary to speak them; therefore, we need not regret them.

LUKE 21

21:1-4 / The Widow's Offering

How encouraging is Jesus' praise of the poor widow to those of us who may be widows or widowers who are poor. His praise affirms that we, too, have the privilege of following his Way of reaching out to the poor. Unlike the rich people who, as Jesus noted, were thoughtlessly contributing what they could spare (perhaps the "loose change in their pockets"), we might, like the poor widow, give deliberately and with care. In fact, we might plan always to share whatever resources we have, no matter how meager they might be.

We might also exercise care in selecting the recipients of our sharing, whether our church or some other group or persons who are in need of help. Ignoring our own poverty, we might seek means to share what little we have by generously giving to those who may be destitute or who may have been impoverished by a recent disaster.

21:34-36 / Exhortation to Watch

At the conclusion of a number of signs that Jesus presented as signaling the destruction of Jerusalem and the end of time, Jesus cautioned, "Be alert at all times, praying that you may have the strength to escape all these things that will take place, and to stand before the Son of Man."

We have all witnessed tragedies that have resulted in deaths, sometimes in deaths of large groups of people; yet it may be difficult for us to realize that we could be involved in tragedies that could take our lives. As repugnant as

such reflection might be to us, we might deliberately reflect on our possible deaths through
tragedy and pray, as Jesus directed, for
strength to "stand before the Son of Man."

While the frail among us are endeavoring
to live well before God and to prepare for death
in prayer and reflection, the world goes on and
catastrophes occur. Somehow we are part of
these happenings and must be concerned
about them.

21:37-38 / Jesus' Last Days

During the time preceding his capture, the
time left in which he could freely determine his
schedule and activities, Jesus spent his days
teaching in the Temple and his nights on the
Mount of Olives. He seemed to feel an urgency
to accomplish his mission in Jerusalem and the
same urgency to spend a large portion of his
time in prayer. He was active to the end.

In determining how he would live his last
days, Jesus is the model for those of us who are
terminally ill and those who are frail. We might
discern what our final mission in life might be
and find encouragement to continue possible
activities, if only that of valuing and cooperat-
ing with our caregivers. Like Jesus, we might

spend long periods of time in whatever prayer is possible in our weakened state. Like Jesus, to the extent that we can, we might share some of our insights with those around us.

The Passion

LUKE 22

22:1-6 / The Conspiracy against Jesus: Judas Betrays Him

As indicated in Acts 2:23,32; 3:14-15; 4:10; 10:39-40; and 1 Corinthians 15:3-4, Christian preaching about Jesus began with the topics of his death and resurrection. The Passion narratives, therefore, were written before other parts of the gospels. All four canonical gospels are basically similar in their Passion narratives. This similarity indicates that the Passion accounts are more historical than are other parts of the gospels.

In Luke's gospel, Satan had left Jesus after the temptation (4:13) and returned now with Judas' betrayal during the Passion. Luke portrays Satan as entering Judas and the work of Satan as beginning with the Passion.

The frail among us who were placed in institutions without having been consulted may have been betrayed, even if the one who made the decision did not intend betrayal and even if the decision was objectively a good one. We (provided we are lucid) have the right to determine our lives and living spaces. Circumstances, such as the selling of our homes by relatives, may render the decision for institutionalization irreversible, and we, like Jesus, must accept what is. Bereft because of the loss of possessions that linked us to our past and loved ones, we might suffer in union with Jesus, betrayed.

22:7-13 / Preparation for the Passover Supper

Luke saw the Last Supper as a paschal rite, a new paschal rite in which the ancient rite found fulfillment. Because it was the last opportunity before his death and because he wished to prepare the apostles for the ensuing period of conflict, Jesus chose to eat the Passover with the apostles.

Precisely because, in a short time, those of us older persons who are frail and are dying may not be with loved ones and/or friends, we might take care to celebrate meaningful events with them as much as possible. We might even celebrate our coming death and resurrection by participating with loved ones in the liturgy and the anointing of the sick. Even though we lack energy, we might expend the extra effort to be present with loved ones and to convey the messages we want to leave with them, just as Jesus carefully left with the apostles the legacy of his last thoughts and teachings. We might see Jesus as present in celebration.

22:14-20 / *The Supper*

Jesus, who came to live among people and to save them, made sure that he would be with them after his death. He did so in a special way through the Eucharist. Through the ages, the church has faithfully fulfilled Jesus' directive, "Do this in remembrance of me," by preserving the essential tradition of Jesus' words and actions at the Last Supper. Nevertheless, whenever situations arose that hampered the faithful from participating in the Eucharist, the church adjusted the accidental traditions. Thus today those of us who are shut-ins may receive the Eucharist frequently through the visits of non-ordained communion ministers. And those of us who are more active may be privileged to be the ministers who bring the Eucharist to others.

How consoling the Eucharist often is to the anxious among us and to the frail! How wonderful that Jesus left this remembrance of himself in communal celebration and that he made himself present and accessible in ordinary and tangible substances! The celebration of the Eucharist has not only brought us close to Jesus but also united us with one another. Though physically separated from our communities, those of us who are frail may experience communion with the church community through the Eucharist.

22:21-23 / Jesus Foretells the Treachery of Judas

Jesus knew that Judas would betray him. Judas was an apostle, one close to Jesus. How sad Jesus must have felt! That the betrayer was helping fulfill what was decreed does not lessen the gravity of the treachery, for Jesus cried, "Woe to that one by whom he is betrayed!"

Sometimes those of us who are frail "know" when family members are planning to institutionalize us without consulting us, let alone facilitating freedom of choice for us. Yet, we may be helpless in terms of affecting the decision and of conveying how hurt we are to loved ones. That Jesus was helpless and probably saddened in the face of betrayal of his life may be consoling.

As we reflect on Judas' tragic betrayal of Jesus, we might reflect also on whether we have been loyal to Jesus through our loyalty to those who have given themselves to us in friendship over the years. Surely we should not allow a difference of opinion or a change in others' goals to cause us in any way to be disloyal. Instead we might forthrightly express our disagreement to our friends even while we remain faithful.

Judas sold Jesus for money. We might examine our own wants and desires and the actions we take to fulfill them. Do we ever sell another person: a frail parent whom we temporarily neglect, an adult child struggling to support a family while we take another month-long tour, the fourth within a year? We might ask Jesus to help us put our desires and what we might sell to secure them into his perspective.

22:24-27 / Who Is the Greatest?

It is in serving that Jesus sees greatness. Those of us who are frail perhaps have learned and accepted the role of Christian service and, for that very reason, may be discouraged that we can no longer serve. What seems worse, some of us must be the recipients of the services of a caregiver. Moreover, we may realize that the caregiver's work is physically very demanding and psychologically without the reward of seeing us improve with caring service. As a result, we may feel guilty.

Viewing the role of Christian service from a new perspective, however, the frail among us might see ourselves as the means whereby the caregiver has an opportunity to serve as Jesus did. To be the means whereby another participates in Jesus' ministry of service is a special, privileged role. In exercising this role, we with sensitivity may facilitate the caregiver's difficult task—by being especially pleasant, cooperative and understanding. Receiving care might even become a joy!

22:31-34 / Jesus Predicts Peter's Denial and Repentance

In facing the realities of his own suffering and death, Jesus was also helping Peter to face the reality of his weakness. Jesus assured Peter, however, that he had prayed for him that Peter's faith might not fail and that Peter in turn might strengthen the other disciples.

When reflecting on our lives, we may experience agonizing guilt in recalling a past time when, overwhelmed, weak, and frightened, we denied Jesus by failing to support a peer who was suffering a grave injustice or by surrendering to betrayal of our own values when under pressure from others. Just as Jesus prayed for Peter that Peter's faith might not fail, so he forgives and strengthens us in our faith when we are filled with remorse.

22:35-38 / A Time of Crisis

When, during the journey to Jerusalem, Jesus instructed the disciples on their mission (Lk 10:4-10), he had told them not to carry luggage and to depend on what people would give them. Now, however, he poignantly noted, the situation has changed. Jesus is considered "among the lawless," and the people will be hostile to his followers. The peaceful, loving Jesus seemed torn, for he even called for swords.

How easy it is for us to follow the "rules of thumb" for living that our parents taught us or that we evolved over the years. Our rules may be based on sound principles and values; but circumstances change and we change. We are never free, therefore, of the responsibility for ongoing discernment of our way of life and of decisions at critical times. Prayerfully reflecting with Jesus on scripture and on our life realities with Jesus, we might frequently engage in the discernment process, asking that Jesus send the Spirit to enlighten us.

22:39-46 / Jesus Prays on The Mount of Olives

As the disciples slept, Jesus prayed that his suffering be removed. Knowing its inevitability, however, he actively accepted it in his prayer, "Not my will but yours be done." His very real agony on the Mount of Olives may have been his growth to acceptance of death. His was real anguish and fear of the unknown in certain death, so that his sweat fell like great drops of blood.

The fact that Jesus experienced the suffering so common to the dying in accepting God's plan for his death is redeeming. Like Jesus, those of us who are terminally ill may pray that our suffering be removed. Like Jesus, we also might strive actively to accept whatever suffering we or caregivers cannot alleviate.

Jesus' fright affirms us when we are dying and therefore frightened. We know that, just as God's angel strengthened Jesus, so God will be with us and will strengthen us.

22:47-62 / *The Arrest*

Betrayed by Judas, Jesus was arrested. Peter, who followed Jesus from a distance, was afraid and denied Jesus—once, twice, three times. Peter denied Jesus, and the other apostles (with the exception of John; see Jn 19:26) kept their distance from Jesus, arrested, suffering, and dying. Yet, Jesus, when abandoned, remembered Peter and turned to look at him.

Jesus' understanding of Peter may enable us, when dying, to understand and even have compassion for our loved ones if they falter or flee when confronted by suffering and dying in the person of their parent, or brother, or sister. Recalling Jesus' compassionate look of forgiveness of Peter, we might help our loved ones to be more comfortable with us when we are dying by conversing about our deaths before we are too weak.

22:63-65 / The Guards Mock Jesus

Jesus, who respected the freedom of the individual person, was seized and placed under guard. The guards treat him as an object of their sport and cruelty. They beat him. They ridiculed him. Because it touched his very identity as prophet and Messiah, their mockery may have been particularly cruel.

We occasionally may endure insults just because we are old or simply because we are in subservient positions, such as that of recipient of care, customer, bill payer, consumer, or patient. We may be highly indignant, and rightly so, that we are the objects of insults, and we may justifiably object to the insults. However, the fact that Jesus was repeatedly subjected to indignities, cruelty, and lack of ordinary human respect during his Passion may strengthen us to live with what we cannot change.

When we are dying, caregivers may handle our bodies as though we were objects. It may be difficult for us to understand, let alone accept, such undignified suffering: somewhere in the mystery of suffering is the understanding that comes through the realization that God endured this kind of suffering himself.

22:66-71 / Jesus before the Sanhedrin

Jesus' reason for coming to earth, his basic purpose, was in his identity as the Christ. He had said he was the Christ; he taught and preached as such. Although he understood the thinking of those who questioned him, it must have pained him that he had not been heard and was not known as the Christ.

Some of us who may have been well known during more active years may find it painful that no one responds when we say our names. The absence of recognition may be especially difficult if we devoted life to helping others. Those of us who have been less well known may, nevertheless, be hurt if we as older persons seem to fade into the background and are not noticed by people around us. Anonymity somehow detracts from our dignity as persons. That Jesus' identity as Christ was not acknowledged may help us to accept anonymity and to realize that, through his incarnation and redemption, Jesus enhanced our dignity.

LUKE 23

23:2-7 / *Jesus before Pilate*

How hard it must have been for Jesus to hear people distorting and misinterpreting his teachings and actions before an outsider like Pilate. This Roman governor had the power to make a decision, but he could not. Instead, he sent Jesus to Herod, perhaps hoping to rid himself of a problem.

During our middle and late-middle years, we may have been highly respected at work, at home, and in our neighborhood and church communities. Those near us may have listened to us, sought our advice, and respected our decisions.

Now that we are older, however, some of us hear our adult children speaking for us or re-interpreting what we say. Our idiosyncrasies, such as absent-mindedness, are now interpreted as signs of failing as we age. Store clerks ignore us or treat us like children. Judgments may be passed on our lives without consulting us or allowing us to make the decisions that are ours. Despite soundness of mind and body, we are condemned to a false stereotype of senility before we are even frail (and most of us never will be irrational).

Totally at the mercy of his captors, Jesus was not allowed to make decisions affecting the last moments of his life. We must persist in exercising our right to determine our lives. However, in union with Jesus, we might need to accept loved ones who make decisions for us which we are powerless to change.

23:8-12 / Jesus before Herod

Herod, wanting to have fun, looked for a miracle from Jesus. Receiving no reply to his questions, he and his guards made their own fun, put a rich cloak on Jesus, and then shunted Jesus back to Pilate.

Herod saw Jesus as an object to provide amusement. In lucid moments, those among us elderly who have Alzheimer's Disease or are senile from other causes may watch or hear our speech and actions providing amusement to family or caregivers who may not intend harm. This amusement, however, may hurt us, who when lucid are too painfully aware of and hor-rified by the loss of control over our own minds and decision-making ability and over bodily functions. Identifying with Jesus and suffering in union with him may be reassuring and strengthening.

23:13-25 / Jesus before Pilate Again

"Crucify him!" These were the words of a Jerusalem mob. Crucifixion was excruciatingly painful and was the death penalty for the lowest of criminals. Pilate knew; he knew Jesus had done no wrong; he said this to the people. Yet, because the mob shouted and insisted, Pilate released the criminal, Barabbas, and condemned Jesus to death by handing him over to the crowd.

We may have reared our children conscientiously and generously. We may have given them assistance with finances and advice to begin their adult lives and offered emergency help in times of crisis. In our years of frailty, some of us may find that our children, now at the beginning of old age, do not respond in our time of need, even though they may say they are available. Instead, our children might expend their efforts in freeing themselves from all care for us. Without investigating to insure good care or involving us in decisions, they may quickly place us in nursing homes. That our own loved children may respond so may be appalling to us. The children's response may seem like condemnation to death, to crucifixion. Union with Jesus who suffered may be our only recourse.

Jesus was *condemned*. The condemnation was unjust. The fundamental sin, however, was not injustice but condemnation in itself; for God's law is one of love, not judgment and condemnation. God loves us, God's children, always and has dignified us in our very being, which God created. Jesus, through suffering his condemnation and death, redeems us from sin, judgment, and condemnation, whether just or unjust, and enhances our dignity as children of God.

As we age and reflect with our children on the past, some of us may hear a son or daughter condemn us because of a decision or act of the past which the children feel harmfully influenced their lives. This hurtful condemnation comes at a time when we perhaps are reviewing our lives and preparing for our own death. Our only and saving recourse is to seek the all-forgiving Jesus and accept his love and reconciliation. At the same time, we might extend that love and understanding to our children, seeking healing for them, while we express our sorrow to them and to Jesus for past wrongs.

23:26-32 / *The Way to Calvary*

Simon from Cyrene was seized and forced to carry Jesus' cross. He may then have shouldered the cross willingly. We do not seek our crosses (nor should we seek suffering, which in itself is not good). But when crosses come to us, we might take care to bear them willingly and patiently and thus to follow Jesus. Jesus is with those of us who carry the cross as caregivers of others. He is our source of strength for our arduous, unrewarding role.

Some of us who consider future frailty may be anxious as a result of observing our own frail parents, for whom we may have cared. Like Simon from Cyrene, we may have been seized by circumstances and forced to carry the cross of caregiver. Like Simon we may have carried our cross faithfully behind Jesus. When we become frail like our parents, Jesus will lead the way again and strengthen us to walk our own way of the cross.

23:33-34 / *The Crucifixion*

The Roman's carried out the sentence and crucified Jesus. Temple authorities and mob organizers must have been pleased, but Jesus said, "Father, forgive them; for they do not know what they are doing."

We may outlive family, friends, and neighbors and find ourselves alone. Because of recent prolonged illnesses and no acquaintances to whom to turn, we may be without food, medicine, and personal care. Frightened, we could be bitter toward new heedless neighbors, distant self-serving landlords, busy clergy and church members, doctors who respond superficially to our urgent calls, and distant relatives. We might ask for the grace to pray with Jesus, "Father, forgive them; for they do not know what they are doing." In so doing, we may be healed of bitterness and, when our time comes, be ready to die in peace.

23:35-38 / *The Crowd Mocks Jesus*

Jesus was dying. Instead of easing his dying and allowing him his hour in peace, the people watched, their leaders jeered, the soldiers mocked, and an inscription nailed above him pronounced, "This is the King of the Jews."

Jesus was king; however, his was not a glorious kingship but the ignominious kingship of the cross.

When we are dying, only doctors or nurses may be with us any length of time. Instead, we may desire the presence of loved family members or dear friends to stand by in the unknown that is death.

At times, we may long for peace in order to prepare for death and Jesus. Instead, we may be connected to machines that are postponing the time of death because our doctors may be overly afraid of being sued as a result of discontinuing life-sustaining machines. That we and our quality of living and dying seem not to be the doctors' main concern may be like a mockery of the very act of dying of old age. In situations devoid of understanding us and our needs, we can only cling to our dying Savior, Jesus.

23:39-43 / The Good Thief

When others were mocking Jesus, one of the thieves crucified with him acknowledged wrong-doing and expressed faith in Jesus by asking for remembrance in the kingdom. Jesus, dying, responded graciously, "Today you will be with me in Paradise."

As we reflect on Jesus crucified, we are drawn like the good thief to acknowledge our own wrong-doing. At times, we may not be sure that decisions we sincerely make correspond to our responsibilities or to our ministry to serve others in love. We can only do our best and express honestly to Jesus our possibly flawed decisions. Jesus' response to the good thief tells us that we may rely on Jesus to forgive totally, to reward our efforts, and to bring us into his kingdom.

As we approach death, we may seek help from Jesus to forgive and put aside rancor toward those with whom we are still not reconciled. We may need to forgive our children, who may have violated Christian and/or cherished family values. We may need to forgive neglectful caregivers and others. Only when we have forgiven all may we be ready to die in peace.

23:44-46 / Jesus' Death

It is incredible that one who lived so well and was so good to others was executed, and executed in the manner reserved for the lowest of criminals of his day. God the Father loved Jesus. He was the Father's Son. How incomprehensible is the mystery of love that accepts the suffering and death of the loved one! Wouk's Jastrow spoke of this mystery exemplified in Job,

> Who is it who in the end of days will force from God the answer from the storm?...will leave the missing piece to God, and praise His name, crying, "The Lord has given, the Lord has taken away: blessed be the name of the Lord"?...Nobody but the sick, plundered skeleton on the ash heap. Nobody but the beloved of God, the worm that lives a few moments and dies, the handful of dirt that has justified creation. Nobody but Job. He is the only answer, if there is one, to the adversary challenge to an Almighty God, if there is One. Job, the stinking Jew (Herman Wouk, *War and Remembrance* [New York: Pocket Books, 1978], 1066).

Somehow, the quality and meaning of life close to death, when we are frail and suffering, is bound up in the meaning of the crucifixion of Jesus, who loved and loves those who broke him, who accepts and loves us, and who died that all might be saved. Though we may at times become irrational, we may somehow participate in a life of quality until death; like the fondled infant who feels contented without knowing why, we may experience a general sense of well being in knowing that we are loved and cared for by our God.

23:47-56 / After Jesus' Death

All seemed finished. As we face the finality of Jesus' death, we ask ourselves whether Jesus' death accomplished its purpose, whether Jesus died in vain.

We recall that Jesus died for us that we might live as he did after death and not die through sin—ours or others'. Jesus came to us to show us the way to live. His Way was the way of love and respect for others, of compassion, of freedom for each person, of reaching out to those in need. As we approach our own deaths, we might examine how we have or have not lived Jesus' Way. In whatever time is left us, we might renew our resolve to live as Jesus did.

All seemed finished. There was only the centurion to say, "Truly, this was an upright man." And then there was Joseph of Arimathaea to claim Jesus' body and place it in a new tomb.

Those of us who have outlived relatives and friends, when dying, may wonder whether anyone will note our absence. We may have witnessed a hasty funeral and realized that no one referred again to the older person who was once among us. We who live alone know that one day a stranger may find us dead and that no one may miss us. The realization that there will be no one to say, "This was an upright person," may devastate us. But dying does open the way to hope and to Jesus.

After the Resurrection

LUKE 24

24:1-12 / The Empty Tomb

Jesus' suffering and death were real, and his dying was incredibly painful. But he rose from the dead! He lives anew!

Our suffering and dying will be real and perhaps difficult. But death opens into resurrection and union with Jesus! Our faith in our eternal destiny may enable us to endure dying. For, as Paul said in Romans 5:7-8,

> Indeed, rarely will anyone die for a
> righteous person—though perhaps for
> a good person someone might
> actually dare to die. But God proves
> his love for us in that while we still
> were sinners Christ died for us.

Faith in the risen Jesus and in our own eternal destiny may strengthen us as we face our own dying. Thus strengthened, we may live fully each remaining day in collaboration with Jesus, who lives, in growing toward fulfillment of our lives. This last effort may be one of reliance on Jesus, for he fills up what is wanting in us who, as death approaches, may be frightened and physically and psychologically weak.

24:13-27 / *The Road to Emmaus*

Jesus approached the two downcast disciples and walked by their sides. Encouraging them to tell him what they are discussing, he listened. Then he asked if Christ did not have to suffer before entering into his glory. After his crucifixion, Jesus spent time with the apostles and disciples, helping them adjust to the startling truth of his resurrection, so that adjustment might help strengthen their faith.

We are grateful that Jesus spent time with the apostles and assured them of his resurrection and triumph over sin, for Jesus assures us of resurrection also. We know that, through Jesus, evil may not dominate but good may triumph. When we are troubled and downcast, Jesus comes to us and walks by our side as he did with the disciples. He encourages us to tell him the important events of our lives and what is troubling us.

As we speak, Jesus listens. As he did with the Emmaus disciples, he enlightens us so that we may find meaning in our past when we reflect on it and in our present life situations. He assists us to preserve continuity between our past and the present, so that we grow in our sense of self-identity. He helps us discern impending decisions, so that we might live his way. We begin to recognize and know Jesus.

24:36-53 / Jesus' Appearance to the Apostles and the Ascension

Jesus' hands and feet bore the marks of the nails. His presence and his suffering could not be denied. We appreciate Jesus' suffering and death and his sensitivity to the apostles' needs to understand, and adjust to, his resurrection. At a time when the apostles were grieving over his death, Jesus was present to them and assured them that he was alive.

Dying may be difficult, but, just as Jesus was with the apostles, so he will be with us in terms of our needs, particularly when we are dying. Jesus will be with us while we live, perhaps in the burden of a severely and chronically ill brother or sister. Conscious of Jesus' presence with us, we may be assured of his supporting and helping love. We may then draw strength from faith in eternal life and

Jesus, for Jesus will open our minds to faith in these mysteries, just as he opened the minds of the apostles to understand the scriptures.

Jesus led the apostles to the outskirts of Bethany, where he was carried up to heaven. The apostles, having worshiped Jesus, returned to Jerusalem, where they continually praised God in the Temple.

Jerusalem

In the Jerusalem of our lives, we enter Jesus' Passion, dying, and resurrection. This is an awesome time for us. Prayerfully, we might reflect: Having reviewed our past, which brought us to the present, what preparation might we now make for death, resurrection, and eternal life with Jesus? We, too, may experience suffering and pain, our own passion. How might we help ourselves to live with hope while suffering? How might we pray in the midst of our passion?

Chapter Five

In Conclusion: A Remarkable Jesus

Luke wrote of Jesus Incarnate, Son of God. He depicted the Son of God, born a helpless infant of a Jewish maiden, Mary, and placed in a manger, where lowly shepherds paid him homage. He wrote of a remarkable Jesus who remembered his heavenly heritage and the vocation entrusted to him to reveal his heavenly Father.

Proclaimed by John the Baptist, Jesus remembered his Jewish heritage when he reached out, helped, and exalted the lowly, the poor, and the oppressed. This remarkable Jesus related with compassion toward those with whom his own people did not associate—lepers, tax collectors, even a Samaritan.

Luke wrote of the remarkable Jesus who, contrary to his contemporary culture, associated freely with women. He wrote of Jesus, who touched and healed women, forgave the sins of a woman because she showed great love, and restored a son to a widow. He included among his followers women who ministered to him, and he told parables with women as characters. In his relationship with women, he demonstrated respect for their dignity, and women, in turn, never wavered in their faithfulness to him, even when men followers faltered.

Luke's gospel is remarkable in its emphasis on the older persons in Jesus' life—Elizabeth and Zechariah, Anna and Simeon, Simon's mother-in-law, the widow of Nain, the father of the prodigal son, and his own mother, Mary.

Led by the Spirit and goal-oriented, this remarkable Jesus steadily pursued his journey to Jerusalem—to the Jerusalem Temple and to his suffering and death in Jerusalem. He boldly cleansed the Temple of the practices that prevented the Temple's being a place of worship of God and a place of prayer.

When teaching the people and his disciples, he told parables that reversed the values and social order of his time and re-aligned values with the horizontal, ordinary people-structured, moral order of the community of love (traditionally called the kingdom of God). When he reached Jerusalem, the end of his life journey, he chose to enter the city riding on a colt, even while his disciples proclaimed him king. He spent much of his time healing people, especially freeing outcasts from the unclean spirits that enchained them. Often he healed in defiance of the Law.

Luke's remarkable Jesus taught and modeled a way of life, a way that the first Christians later strove to live. Following John the Baptist, he urged the people to repentance and promised that forgiveness of sins would ensue. He retreated to the desert for forty days and frequently, probably daily, retreated from active engagement with others in order to pray.

He taught love of others, including non-Jews, and assured the people of the extraordinary love and mercy of God for them, even when they sinned. When he knew that his Passion and death were imminent, he celebrated the Passover meal with the apostles and remarkably and sensitively left a memorial for them—the Eucharist, which even today unites us to him.

That this remarkable Jesus, who taught and modeled love of the lowly and despised and love of enemies, suffered and died as the lowest of criminals is perhaps the most mystifying event of his life. The horrendousness of the event is mitigated wondrously and only by the life-giving hope instilled by his resurrection and ascension. This hope extended to the hope of eventual resurrection for all of his followers.

We Remarkable Older Followers

No one else in the course of history has so dignified each person without exception as has Jesus, the promised one of the Father. Moreover, he has dignified every stage of human life, including our gradual, and perhaps longed-for, dying, with its accompanying gradual deterioration of the body and sometimes of the mind, and with the loss of all else. For death, however difficult, is the means of releasing us from a spent body and mind to resurrection and life eternal with Jesus.

Every stage of our lives, then, is intended to be lived to the full, to be lived according to the example and teachings of Jesus. Our older years have become, through Jesus, that stage which is closest to the goal of life: resurrection and eternal life.

As older persons, we truly decline and die; but then we just as truly live. Like the apostles, some of whom Jesus called from the vocation of fishermen to the vocation of fishers of persons, we are called to a "new" vocation in our older years. Exercising our "generative" responsibility to society, we seek ways to share with others the wisdom we have gained in life. Even while we experience decline, spiritually we are called to integrity, to becoming more and more authentically *person*, more authentically the unique persons whom God created. The closer we are to death and resurrection, the more urgent is our call.

Just as Luke's Jesus remembered scripture and the prophets as foretelling his mission, death, and resurrection, so we remember and review the past and the ways God was with us during our journey through life. We, in remembering, repent of past sins, reconcile self with those whom we have offended and whom we can reach, and attain the peace of the guiltless, knowing that Jesus forgives those who love him.

Just as Jesus took his life, as it was, and offered it to the Father during his shameful crucifixion, so we, having reviewed our past lives, accept our lives in their uniqueness, in their grandeur and non-grandeur, and offer them to the Father in whatever kind of death awaits us. We do so with a sense of dignity and self-worth stemming from creation by God, from Jesus' love and response to the persons of his time, and from the assurance of Jesus' love for us.

While remembering our own histories, we confront a present or a near future that may be fraught with illness and pain. The future may require some of the most drastic changes of our lives. These changes may uproot us, who have already lost family and friends in death. The changes may destroy continuity with the past and result in disorientation and depression.

This plight or the dread of it may provoke us, like Jesus, to cry out in anguish, "Father,... remove this cup from me" (Lk 22:42). With this cry we may sink into the depths of depression and a crisis of faith. If, even when assaulted by doubt, we can cling to Jesus so anguished, we will emerge from the faith crisis with increased growth and depth of faith. We will finally accept what cannot be changed in union with Jesus: "Yet, not my will but yours be done" (Lk 22:42). Surely the Jesus who walked through the countryside, who had nowhere to lay his head, who anguished during the agony in the garden, and who was suddenly pulled away during his Passion from his daily routine of prayer—surely this Jesus will be with us and will be the source of our strength, comfort, and spiritual growth.

In the light of the Lucan-Jesus message, of Jesus' Way, and of the evaluation and perspective gained through reflection on our lives, we acknowledge the values that have influenced us in the past. Prayerfully and reflectively, we clarify the values that are important to us in the remaining years, and strive for a re-ordering of life according to these values.

Valuing those with whom we are in contact, we exert the energy to foster good relationships as well as love and concern for these others. We muster whatever energy is ours to minister to those in need, particularly the oppressed and the poor. Valuing self, we will to make the personal decisions that enable following Jesus. If nothing else is possible for us, we simply make that final choice, the choice of faith in Jesus to the end.

For Our Autumn Years

As we bring to closure our reflections on Jesus' message through Luke, we may wish to bring with us some considerations that may need further development. Knowing that God's call to us is always renewed, we might re-visit our "vocation" discernments to ask ourselves what we discern as God's call to us now. As far as we can determine, to what kind of life does God call us in our still older years?

Do we have "unfinished business" to take care of in this, the last stage of our lives: reconciliation with someone from whom we have been alienated; some messages we want to convey to family members; about our last will and testament; or even our memorial liturgy? Are there changes we might make in our daily living in order to be in ever more prayerful union with our God now and for all eternity?

Finally, there is one last reflection.

In Autumn

Picture yourself sitting on a bench in a park that has many trees. It is October. Some trees, those that do not shed leaves, are a solid, strong green. The leaves of those trees that shed leaves have changed color. Imagine the array of colors. A gentle breeze is blowing. Every so often a leaf floats through the breeze to the ground. Feel yourself in this setting.

After a time, you look up. Someone is coming toward you. As the person approaches, you think you may know him. The person comes to your bench. With a leap of your heart, you realize this is someone very important to you. Then you know. It is Jesus! You watch breathlessly as Jesus picks up a fallen maple leaf. With a smile, he greets you and asks to sit with you.

He begins to talk about the leaf—how it was once hanging on a strong young maple tree. It was green then; water flowed from the tree into its veins. Jesus points to the beauty of the leaf now, to the variety of colors in it—from green to red—even to the withered, crisp edges. He turns to you and says,

"You are more beautiful than this leaf. I remember when you came to know me. You began to talk to me and we became friends. You were young then. There were heartaches—and joys. I remember the people for whom you cared and the hard work you accomplished. I was so proud of you!

"Now you can look back on those years and be proud of them. But now, even more, you have time to talk to me and to listen. You have time for other persons, time to think, time to live and be yourself."

Index of Scripture References

Index of Topics

The topics in this index are from reflections concerning older persons, not fromscripture passages regarding Luke or Jesus.